Oral medicine
Update for the dental practitioner

Crispian Scully CBE
Professor, Consultant and Dean
Eastman Dental Institute University College London
256, Gray's Inn Road, London, WC1X 8LD
UK

Adjunct Professor
Institute of Dentistry
University of Helsinki
Helsinki, FIN-00014
Finland

David H Felix
Consultant and Honorary Clinical Senior Lecturer
Glasgow Dental Hospital and School
378, Sauchiehall Street, Glasgow, G2 3JZ
UK

Associate Dean for Postgraduate Dental Education
NHS Education for Scotland
2nd Floor, Hanover Buildings, 66, Rose Street, Edinburgh, EH2 2NN
UK

2006
Published by the British Dental Association
64 Wimpole Street, London, W1G 8YS

Preface

This book has been developed from a series written for the *British Dental Journal* and provides an overview of current thinking in the more relevant areas of oral medicine for primary care practitioners, written by the authors while they were holding the Presidencies of the European Association for Oral Medicine and the British Society for Oral Medicine, respectively. It includes additionally, a chapter on Human Immunodeficiency Virus infection and a bibliography.

The book gives the detail necessary to assist the primary dental clinical team caring for patients with oral complaints that may be seen in general dental practice. Space precludes inclusion of illustrations of uncommon or rare disorders, or discussion of disorders affecting the hard tissues. Approaching the subject mainly by the symptomatic approach, as it largely relates to the presenting complaint, was considered to be a more helpful approach for GDPs rather than taking a diagnostic category approach.

The clinical aspects of the relevant disorders are discussed, including a brief overview of the aetiology, detail on the clinical features and how the diagnosis is made. Guidance on management and when to refer is also provided, along with relevant websites which offer further detail.

Crispian Scully CBE
David H Felix

Edinburgh, Glasgow and London
May, 2006

ISBN 0 904588 89 0

Printed and bound by
Dennis Barber Limited, Lowestoft, Suffolk

Contents

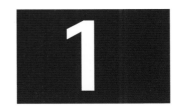

Aphthous and other common ulcers

Specialist referral may be indicated if the practitioner feels:
- the diagnosis is unclear
- a serious diagnosis is possible
- systemic disease may be present
- unclear as to investigations indicated
- complex investigations unavailable in primary care are indicated
- unclear as to treatment indicated
- treatment is complex
- treatment requires agents not readily available
- unclear as to the prognosis
- the patient wishes this.

ULCERATION

Ulceration is a breach in the oral epithelium, which typically exposes nerve endings in the underlying lamina propria, resulting in pain or soreness, especially when eating spicy foods or citrus fruits. Patients vary enormously in the degree to which they suffer and complain of soreness in relation to oral ulceration. It is always important to exclude serious disorders such as oral cancer (Chapter 9) or other serious disease, but not all patients who complain of soreness have discernible organic disease. Conversely, some with serious disease have no pain. Even in those with detectable lesions, the level of complaint can vary enormously. Some patients with large ulcers complain little; others with minimal ulceration complain bitterly of discomfort. Sometimes there is a psychogenic influence.

Terminology

Epithelial thinning or breaches may be seen in:
- **mucosal atrophy or desquamation** – terms often used for thinning of the epithelium which assumes a red appearance as the underlying lamina propria containing blood vessels shows

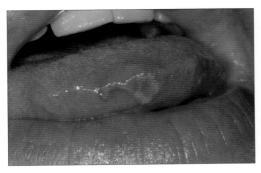

Fig. 1 A small erosion

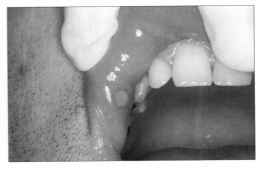

Fig. 2 Minor aphthous ulcer, labial mucosa

through. Most commonly this is seen in desquamative gingivitis (usually related to lichen planus, or less commonly to pemphigoid) and in geographic tongue (erythema migrans or benign migratory glossitis). A similar process may also be seen in systemic disorders such as deficiency states (of iron, folic acid or B vitamins).

- **mucosal inflammation** (mucositis, stomatitis) - which can cause soreness. Viral stomatitis, candidosis, radiation mucositis, chemotherapy-related mucositis and graft-versus-host-disease are examples.
- **erosion** - which is the term used for superficial breaches of the epithelium. These often have a red appearance initially as there is little damage to the underlying lamina propria, but they typically become covered by a fibrinous exudate which has a yellowish appearance (Fig. 1). Erosions are common in vesiculobullous disorders such as pemphigoid.
- **ulcer** - which is the term usually used where there is damage both to epithelium and lamina propria. An inflammatory halo, if present, also highlights the ulcer with a red halo around the yellow or grey ulcer (Fig. 2). Most ulcers are due to local causes such as trauma or burns, but recurrent aphthous stomatitis and cancer must always be considered.

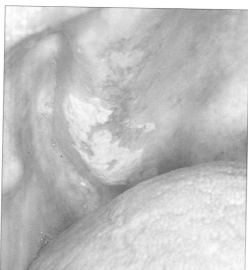

Fig. 3 Chemical burn, right maxillary tuberosity

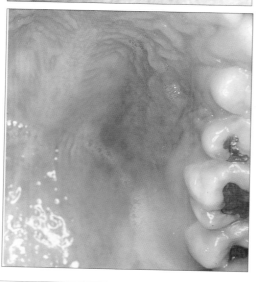

Fig. 4 Thermal burn, palate

Table 1 Main causes of oral ulceration

Local causes
Aphthae
Infections
Drugs
Malignant disease
Systemic diseases

Table 2 Main causes of mouth ulcers

Local causes
Trauma
    Appliances
    Iatrogenic
    Non-accidental injury
    Self-inflicted
    Sharp teeth or restorations
Burns
    Chemical
    Cold
    Electric
    Heat
    Radiation
Recurrent aphthae
Infections
    Acute necrotising gingivitis
    Chickenpox
    Deep mycoses
    Hand, foot and mouth disease
    Herpangina
    Herpetic stomatitis
    HIV
    Infectious mononucleosis
    Syphilis
    Tuberculosis
    Zoster
Drugs
    Cytotoxic drugs,
    Nicorandil, NSAIDs
    Beta blockers
    Many others
Malignant neoplasms
    Oral
    Encroaching from antrum
Systemic disease
Mucocutaneous disease
    Behçet's syndrome
    Chronic ulcerative stomatitis
    Epidermolysis bullosa
    Erythema multiforme
    Lichen planus
    Pemphigus vulgaris
    Sub-epithelial immune blistering diseases
    (Pemphigoid and variants, dermatitis
    herpetiformis, linear IgA disease)
Haematological disorders
    Anaemia
    Gammopathies
    Haematinic deficiencies
    Leukaemia and myelodysplastic syndrome
    Neutropenia and other white cell dyscrasias
Gastrointestinal disease
    Coeliac disease
    Crohn's disease
    Ulcerative colitis
Miscellaneous uncommon diseases
    Eosinophilic ulcer
    Giant cell arteritis
    Hypereosinophilic syndrome
    Lupus erythematosus
    Necrotising sialometaplasia
    Periarteritis nodosa
    Reiters syndrome
    Sweet's syndrome
    Wegener's granulomatosis

Causes of oral ulceration

Ulcers and erosions can also be the final common manifestation of a spectrum of conditions. These range from: epithelial damage resulting from trauma; an immunological attack as in lichen planus, pemphigoid or pemphigus; damage because of an immune defect as in HIV disease and leukaemia; infections such as herpesviruses, tuberculosis and syphilis; cancer and nutritional defects such as vitamin deficiencies and some gastrointestinal diseases (Tables 1 and 2).

Ulcers of local causes

At any age, there may be burns from chemicals of various kinds (Fig. 3), heat (Fig. 4), cold, or ionising radiation or factitious ulceration, especially of the maxillary gingivae or palate.

Children may develop ulceration of the lower lip by accidental biting following dental local anaesthesia. Ulceration of the upper labial fraenum, especially in a child with bruised and swollen lips, subluxed teeth or fractured jaw can represent non-accidental injury. At any age, trauma, hard foods, or appliances may also cause ulceration. The lingual fraenum may be traumatised by repeated rubbing over the lower incisor teeth in cunnilingus, in recurrent coughing as in whooping cough, or in self-mutilating conditions.

Most ulcers of local cause have an obvious aetiology, are acute, usually single ulcers, last less than three weeks and heal spontaneously. Chronic trauma may produce an ulcer with a keratotic margin (Fig. 5).

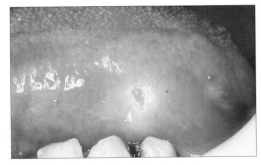

Fig. 5 Traumatic ulceration, lateral tongue

Recurrent aphthous stomatitis (RAS; aphthae; canker sores)

RAS is a very common condition which typically starts in childhood or adolescence and presents with multiple recurrent small, round or ovoid ulcers with circumscribed margins, erythematous haloes, and yellow or grey floors (Figs. 2 and 6).

RAS affects at least 20% of the population, with the highest prevalence in higher socio-economic classes. Virtually all dentists will see patients with aphthae.

Aetiopathogenesis

Immune mechanisms appear at play in a person with a genetic predisposition to oral ulceration. There is a positive family history in about one third of patients with RAS. Immunological factors are also involved, with T helper cells predominating in the RAS lesions early on, along with some

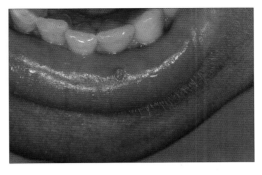

Fig. 6 Minor aphthous ulceration

natural killer (NK) cells. Cytotoxic cells then appear in the lesions and there is evidence for an antibody dependent cellular cytotoxicity (ADCC) reaction. It now seems likely therefore that a minor degree of immunological dysregulation underlies aphthae.

RAS may be a group of disorders of different pathogeneses. Cross-reacting antigens between the oral mucosa and microorganisms may be the initiators, but attempts to implicate a variety of bacteria or viruses have failed.

Predisposing factors

Most people who suffer RAS are otherwise apparently completely well. In a few, predisposing factors may be identifiable, or suspected. These include:

1. Stress: underlies RAS in many cases. RAS are typically worse at examination times.
2. Trauma: biting the mucosa, and dental appliances may lead to some aphthae.
3. Haematinic deficiency (deficiencies of iron, folic acid (folate) or vitamin B_{12}) in up to 20% of patients.
4. Sodium lauryl sulphate (SLS), a detergent in some oral healthcare products may produce oral ulceration.
5. Cessation of smoking: may precipitate or aggravate RAS.
6. Gastrointestinal disorders particularly coeliac disease (gluten-sensitive enteropathy) and Crohn's disease in about 3% of patients.
7. Endocrine factors in some women whose RAS are clearly related to the fall in progestogen level in the luteal phase of their menstrual cycle.
8. Immune deficiency: ulcers similar to RAS may be seen in HIV and other immune defects.
9. Food allergies: underlie RAS rarely.

Drugs may produce aphthous-like lesions (see below).

Key points for dentists: aphthous ulcers

- They are so common that all dentists will see them
- It is important to rule out predisposing causes (sodium lauryl sulphate, certain foods/drinks, stopping smoking or vitamin or other deficiencies) or conditions such as Behçet's syndrome
- Enquire about eye, genital, gastrointestinal or skin lesions
- Topical corticosteroids are the main treatment

Clinical features

There are three main clinical types of RAS, though the significance of these distinctions is unclear and it is conceivable that they may represent three different diseases:

1. Minor aphthous ulcers (MiAU; Mikulicz Ulcer) occur mainly in the 10 to 40-year-old age group, often cause minimal symptoms, and are small round or ovoid ulcers 2-4 mm in diameter. The ulcer floor is initially yellowish but assumes a greyish hue as healing and epithelialisation proceeds. They are surrounded by an erythematous halo and some oedema, and are found mainly on the non-keratinised mobile mucosa of the lips, cheeks, floor of the mouth, sulci or ventrum of the tongue. They are only uncommonly seen on the keratinised mucosa of the palate or dorsum of the tongue and occur in groups of only a few ulcers (one to six) at a time. They heal in seven to 10 days, and recur at intervals of one to four months leaving little or no evidence of scarring (Fig. 7).

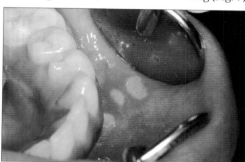

Fig. 7 Minor aphthae

2. Major aphthous ulcers (MjAU; Sutton's Ulcers; periadenitis mucosa necrotica recurrens (PMNR)) (Figs 8 and 9) are larger, of longer duration, of more frequent recurrence, and often more painful than minor ulcers. MjAU are round or ovoid like minor ulcers, but they are larger and associated with surrounding oedema and can reach a large size, usually about 1 cm in diameter or even larger. They

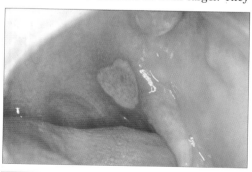

Fig. 8 Major aphthous ulceration, soft palate complex

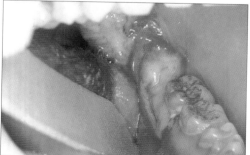

Fig. 9 Major aphthous ulceration

are found on any area of the oral mucosa, including the keratinised dorsum of the tongue or palate, occur in groups of only a few ulcers (one to six) at one time and heal slowly over 10 to 40 days. They recur extremely frequently, may heal with scarring and are occasionally found with a raised erythrocyte sedimentation rate or plasma viscosity.

3. Herpetiform Ulceration (HU) is found in a slightly older age group than the other forms of RAS and mainly in females. They begin with vesiculation which passes rapidly into multiple minute pinhead-sized discrete ulcers (Fig. 10), which involve any oral site including the keratinised mucosa. They increase in size and coalesce to leave large round ragged ulcers, which heal in 10 days or longer, are often extremely painful and recur so frequently that ulceration may be virtually continuous.

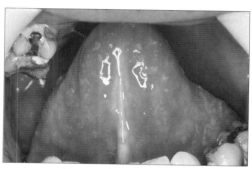

Fig. 10 Herpetiform aphthae

Diagnosis

Specific tests are unavailable, so the diagnosis must be made on history and clinical features alone. However, to exclude the systemic disorders discussed above, it is often useful to undertake the investigations shown in Table 3. Biopsy is rarely indicated, and only when a different diagnosis is suspected.

Table 3 Investigation of aphthae
Full blood count
Haematinics
Ferritin
Folate
Vitamin B_{12}
Screen for coeliac disease

Management

Other similar disorders such as Behçet's syndrome must be ruled out (see below). Predisposing factors should then be corrected. Fortunately, the natural history of RAS is one of eventual remission in most cases. However, few patients do not have spontaneous remission for several years and although there is no curative treatment, measures should be taken to relieve symptoms, correct reversible causes (haematological disorder, trauma) and reduce ulcer duration.

Maintain good oral hygiene

Chlorhexidine or triclosan mouthwashes may help.

Table 4 Examples of readily available topical corticosteroids

Steroid	UK trade name	Dosage every six hours
Low potency		
Hydrocortisone hemisuccinate pellets	Corlan	2.5 mg pellet dissolved in mouth close to ulcers
Medium potency		
Triamcinolone acetonide 0.1% in carmellose gelatin paste	Adcortyl in Orabase	Apply paste to dried lesions
Betamethasone phosphate tablets	Betnesol	0.5 mg; use as mouthwash
High potency		
Beclometasone (Beclomethasone) dipropionate spray	Becotide 100	1 puff (100 micrograms) to lesions

There is a spectrum of topical anti-inflammatory agents that may help in the management of RAS.

Topical corticosteroids can usually control symptoms

Common preparations used include the following, four times daily:

- Weak potency corticosteroids - topical hydrocortisone hemisuccinate pellets (Corlan), 2.5 mg
or
- Medium potency steroids - topical triamcinolone acetonide in carboxymethyl cellulose paste (Adcortyl in Orabase), or betamethasone (Betnesol)
or
- Higher potency topical corticosteroids (eg beclometasone) (Table 4).

The major concern is adrenal suppression with long-term and/or repeated application, but there is evidence that 0.05% fluocinonide in adhesive paste and betamethasone-17-valerate mouthrinse do not cause this problem.

Topical tetracycline (eg doxycycline), or tetracycline plus nicotinamide may provide relief and reduce ulcer duration, but should be avoided in children under 12 who might ingest the tetracycline and develop tooth staining and in breast feeding. If RAS fails to respond to these measures, systemic immunomodulators may be required, under specialist supervision.

Key points for patients: aphthous ulcers

- These are common
- They are not thought to be infectious
- Children may inherit ulcers from parents
- The cause is not known but some follow use of toothpaste with sodium lauryl sulphate, certain foods/drinks, or stopping smoking
- Some vitamin or other deficiencies or conditions may predispose to ulcers
- Ulcers can be controlled but rarely cured
- No long-term consequences are known

Websites and patient information

http://www.usc.edu/hsc/dental/opath/Cards/Ap hthousStomatitis.html
http://openseason.com/annex/library/cic/X003 3_fever.txt.html

Infections

Infections that cause mouth ulcers are mainly viral, especially the herpesviruses, Coxsackie, ECHO and HIV viruses. Bacterial causes of mouth ulcers, apart from acute necrotising ulcerative gingivitis, are less common. Syphilis and tuberculosis are uncommon but increasing, especially in people with HIV/AIDS. Fungal and protozoal causes of ulcers are also uncommon but increasingly seen in immunocompromised persons, and travellers from the developing world.

Herpes simplex virus (HSV)

The term 'herpes' is often used loosely to refer to infections with herpes simplex virus (HSV). This is a ubiquitous virus which commonly produces lesions in the mouth and oropharynx. HSV is contracted by close contact with infected individuals from infected saliva or other body fluids after an incubation period of approximately four to seven days.

Primary infection is often subclinical between the ages of 2-4 years but may present with stomatitis (gingivostomatitis). This is usually caused by HSV-1 and is commonly attributed to 'teething' particularly if there is a fever. In teenagers or older people, this may be due to HSV-2 transmitted sexually. Generally speaking, HSV infections above the belt (oral or oropharyngeal) are caused by HSV-1 but below the belt (genital or anal) are caused by HSV-2.

The mouth or oropharynx is sore (herpetic stomatitis or gingivostomatitis): there is a single episode of oral vesicles which may be widespread, and which break down to leave oral ulcers that are initially pin-point but fuse to produce irregular painful ulcers. Gingival oedema, erythema and ulceration are prominent, the cervical lymph nodes may be enlarged and tender, and there is sometimes fever and/or malaise. Patients with immune defects are liable to severe and/or protracted infections.

HSV is neuroinvasive and neurotoxic and infects neurones of the dorsal root and autonomic ganglia. HSV remains latent thereafter in those ganglia, usually the trigeminal ganglion, but can be reactivated to result in clinical recrudescence (see below).

Diagnosis

Diagnosis is largely clinical. Viral studies are used occasionally and can include:

- culture; this takes days to give a result
- electron microscopy; this is not always available
- polymerase chain reaction (PCR) detection of HSV-DNA; this is sensitive but expensive
- immunodetection; detection of HSV antigens is of some value.

Management

Although patients have spontaneous healing within 10-14 days, treatment is indicated particularly to reduce fever and control pain. Adequate fluid intake is important, especially in children, and antipyretics/analgesics such as paracetamol/acetoaminophen elixir help. A soft bland diet may be needed, as the mouth can be very sore. Aciclovir orally or parenterally is useful mainly in immunocompromised patients or in the otherwise apparently healthy patient if seen early in the course of the disease but does not reduce the frequency of subsequent recurrences.

Recurrent HSV infections

Up to 15% of the population have recurrent HSV-1 infections, typically on the lips (herpes labialis: cold sores) from reactivation of HSV latent in the trigeminal ganglion. The virus is shed into saliva, and there may be clinical recrudescence. Reactivating factors include fever such as caused by upper respiratory tract infection (hence herpes labialis is often termed 'cold' sores), sunlight, menstruation, trauma and immunosuppression.

Lip lesions at the mucocutaneous junction may be preceded by pain, burning, tingling or itching. Lesions begin as macules that rapidly become papular, then vesicular for about 48 hours, then pustular, and finally scab within 72-96 hours and heal without scarring (Fig. 11).

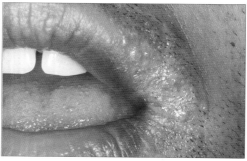

Fig. 11 Herpes labialis

Recurrent intraoral herpes in apparently healthy patients tends to affect the hard palate or gingivae with a small crop of ulcers which heals within one to two weeks. Lesions are usually over the greater palatine foramen, following a palatal local anaesthetic injection, presumably because of the trauma.

Recurrent intraoral herpes in immunocompromised patients may appear as chronic, often dendritic, ulcers, often on the tongue.

Diagnosis

Diagnosis is largely clinical; viral studies are used occasionally.

Management

Most patients will have spontaneous remission within one week to 10 days but the condition is both uncomfortable and unsightly, and thus treatment is indicated. Antivirals will achieve maximum benefit only if given early in the disease but may be indicated in patients who have severe, widespread or persistent lesions and in immunocompromised persons. Lip lesions in healthy patients may be minimised with penciclovir 1% cream or aciclovir 5% cream applied in the prodrome. In immunocompromised patients, systemic aciclovir or other antivirals such as valaciclovir (the precursor of penciclovir) may be needed.

Websites and patient information

http://www.mayoclinic.com/health/cold-sore/D500358

Key points for patients: cold sores
- These are common
- They are caused by a virus (Herpes simplex) which lives in nerves forever
- They are infectious and the virus can be transmitted by kissing
- They may be precipitated by sun-exposure, stress, injury or immune problems
- They have no long-term consequences
- They may be controlled by antiviral creams or tablets, best used *early* on

Drug-induced ulceration

Drugs may induce ulcers by producing a local burn, or by a variety of mechanisms such as the induction of lichenoid lesions (Fig. 12). Cytotoxic drugs (eg methotrexate) commonly produce ulcers, but non-steroidal anti-inflammatory drugs (NSAIDs), beta blockers alendronate (a bisphosphonate), nicorandil (a cardiac drug) and a range of other drugs may also cause ulcers.

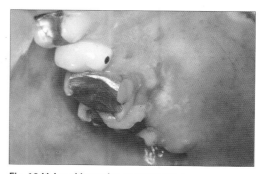

Fig. 12 Lichenoid reaction to propranolol

A drug history is important to elicit such uncommon reactions, and then the offending drug should be avoided.

Patients to refer:
- Severe aphthae
- Malignancy
- HIV-related ulceration
- TB or syphilis
- Drug-related ulceration
- Systemic disease.

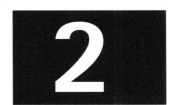

Mouth ulcers of more serious connotation

MALIGNANT ULCERS

A range of neoplasms may present with ulcers; most commonly these are carcinomas (Fig. 1), but Kaposi's sarcoma, lymphomas and other neoplasms may be seen and are discussed in Article 9. Most present with a single persistent ulcer. Biopsy is usually required to establish the diagnosis.

SYSTEMIC DISEASE

A wide range of systemic diseases, especially mucocutaneous diseases, blood, gut, and miscellaneous uncommon disorders, may cause oral lesions which, because of the moisture, trauma and infection in the mouth, tend to break down to leave ulcers or erosions. Most present with multiple often persistent ulcers. Biopsy is often required to establish the diagnosis.

MUCOCUTANEOUS DISORDERS

Mucocutaneous disease that may cause oral erosions or ulceration (or occasionally blisters) include particularly Behcet's syndrome, and a number of skin diseases including lichen planus (Fig. 2; see Article 5), occasionally erythema multiforme or pemphigoid, and rarely pemphigus.

BEHÇET'S SYNDROME

Behçet's syndrome (BS) is a rare condition. It is the association of recurrent mouth ulcers with genital ulceration and eye disease, but other systemic manifestations may also be seen. The disease is found worldwide, but most commonly in people from Eastern Mediterranean countries (particularly Greeks, Turks, Arabs and Jews) and along the Silk Route taken by Marco Polo across eastern Asia, China, Korea and Japan.

Aetiopathogenesis

Behçet's syndrome is a vasculitis that has not been proved to be infectious, contagious or

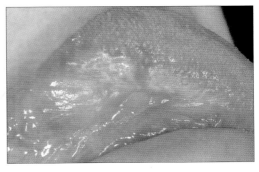

Fig. 1 Squamous cell carcinoma

Fig. 2 Lichen planus

sexually transmitted. There are many immunological findings in BS similar to those seen in recurrent aphthous stomatitis, with T suppressor cell dysfunction and increased polymorphonuclear leucocyte motility (Article 1). There is a genetic predisposition. Many of the features of BS (erythema nodosum, arthralgia, uveitis) are common to established immune complex diseases.

Clinical features

Behçet's syndrome is a chronic, sometimes life-threatening disorder characterised mainly by:

- Recurrent mouth ulcers in 90–100%
- Recurrent painful genital ulcers that tend to heal with scars
- Ocular lesions: iridocyclitis, uveitis, retinal vascular changes, and optic atrophy may occur
- CNS lesions
- Skin lesions: erythema nodosum, papulopustular lesions and acneiform nodules.

The joints, epididymis, heart, intestinal tract, vascular system and most other systems may also be involved.

However, very non-specific signs and symptoms, which may be recurrent, may precede the onset of the mucosal ulcerations by six months to five years.

Differential diagnosis

This is from a range of other syndromes that can affect the eyes, mouth and skin – such as various dermatological disorders and infections.

Diagnosis

BS can be very difficult to diagnose, but the International Study Group for Behçet's Disease (ISGBD) criteria suggest the diagnosis be made on clinical grounds alone on the basis of recurrent mouth ulcers plus two or more of the following:

- Recurrent genital ulceration
- Eye lesions
- Skin lesions
- Pathergy – a >2 mm diameter erythematous nodule or pustule forming 24–48 hours after sterile subcutaneous puncture of the forearm.

Investigations

There is no specific diagnostic test, but typing for specific human leukocyte antigens (HLA B5101) can help. Disease activity may be assessed by serum levels of various proteins, such as the erythrocyte sedimentation rate (ESR) and C-reactive protein (CRP) or antibodies to intermediate filaments.

Management

In the face of the difficult diagnosis and serious potential complications, patients with suspected BS should be referred early for specialist advice.

Websites and patient information

http://www.aarda.org/indexf.html

LICHEN PLANUS

Lichen planus is discussed in Chapter 5.

ERYTHEMA MULTIFORME

Erythema multiforme (EM) is an uncommon acute often recurrent reaction affecting mucocutaneous tissues, seen especially in younger males.

The aetiology is unclear in most patients, but it appears to be an immunological hypersensitivity reaction, leading to sub- and intra-epithelial vesiculation. There may be a genetic predisposition with associations of recurrent EM with various HLA haplotypes.

EM is triggered by a range of usually exogenous factors, such as:

- Infective agents , particularly HSV (herpes-associated EM: HAEM) and the bacterium *Mycoplasma pneumoniae*
- Drugs such as sulfonamides (e.g. co-trimoxazole), cephalosporins, aminopenicillins, and many others
- Food additives or chemicals.

Clinical features

EM ranges from limited disease (Minor EM) to severe, widespread life-threatening illness (Major EM). Most patients (70%) in either form, have oral lesions, which may precede lesions on other stratified squamous epithelia (eyes, genitals or skin), or may arise in isolation. Oral EM typically presents with macules which evolve to blisters and ulcers. The lips become swollen, cracked, bleeding and crusted.

Minor EM affects only one site and may affect mouth alone, or skin or other mucosae. Rashes are various but typically 'iris' or 'target' lesions or bullae on extremities.

Major EM (Stevens-Johnson syndrome; SJS) almost invariably involves the oral mucosa and causes widespread lesions affecting mouth, eyes, pharynx, larynx, oesophagus, skin and genitals.

Diagnosis

There are no specific diagnostic tests for EM. Therefore, the diagnosis is mainly clinical, and it can be difficult to differentiate between it and viral stomatitis, pemphigus, toxic epidermal necrolysis, and sub-epithelial immune blistering disorders. Serology for HSV or *Mycoplasma pneumoniae*, or other micro-organisms, and biopsy of perilesional tissue, with histological and immunostaining examination, are essential if a specific diagnosis is required.

Management

Spontaneous healing can be slow – up to two to three weeks in minor EM and up to six weeks in major EM.

Treatment is therefore indicated but controversial and thus specialist care should be sought. Supportive care is important; a liquid diet and even intravenous fluid therapy may be necessary. Oral hygiene should be improved with 0.2% aqueous chlorhexidine mouthbaths.

The use of corticosteroids is controversial but minor EM may respond to topical corticosteroids. Patients with major EM such as the Stevens-Johnson syndrome may need to be admitted for hospital care. Major EM patients should be referred for treatment with systemic corticosteroids or other immunomodulatory drugs.

Websites and patient information
http://www.emedicine.com/EMERG/topic173.htm

PEMPHIGOID
Pemphigoid is the term given to a group of uncommon sub-epithelial immunologically-mediated vesiculobullous disorders (SEIMD) which can affect stratified squamous epithelium, characterised by damage to one of the protein constituents of the basement membrane zone (BMZ) anchoring filaments components. A number of other sub-epithelial vesiculobullous disorders may produce similar clinical features (Table 1).

Table 1 Sub-epithelial vesiculobullous disorders
Pemphigoid variants
Acquired epidermolysis bullosa (EBA)
Toxic epidermal necrolysis (TEN)
Erythema multiforme
Dermatitis herpetiformis
Linear IgA disease
Chronic bullous dermatosis of childhood

The main types of pemphigoid that involve the mouth are:
- Mucous membrane pemphigoid (MMP), in which mucosal lesions predominate but skin lesions are rare
- Oral mucosal pemphigoid — patients with oral lesions only, without a progressive ocular scarring process and without serologic reactivity to bullous pemphigoid (BP) antigens
- Bullous pemphigoid (BP) — which affects mainly the skin
- Ocular pemphigoid — which is sometimes termed cicatricial pemphigoid (CP) since it may cause serious conjunctival scarring.

However, most of the literature has failed to distinguish these variants, since their distinction has only recently been recognised, and therefore the following discussion groups them together.

MUCOUS MEMBRANE/ORAL PEMPHIGOID
Mucous membrane pemphigoid (benign mucous membrane pemphigoid) is an uncommon chronic disease, twice as common in females, and usually presenting in the fifth to sixth decades.

Mucous membrane pemphigoid is an autoimmune type of disorder with a genetic predisposition. The precipitating event is unclear in most cases, but rare cases are drug-induced (eg by furosemide or penicillamine). It is characterised immunologically by deposition of IgG and C3 antibodies directed against the epithelial basement membrane zone (BMZ). There are also circulating autoantibodies to BMZ components present in hemi-desmosomes or the lamina lucida.

The antibodies damage the BMZ and histologically there is a sub-basilar split. The pathogenesis probably includes complement-mediated sequestration of leukocytes with resultant cytokine and leukocyte enzyme release and detachment of the basal cells from the BMZ.

Clinical features
The oral lesions (Figs 3–5) affect especially the gingivae and palate, and include bullae or vesicles which are tense, may be blood-filled and remain intact for several days. Persistent irregular erosions or ulcers appear after the blisters burst and, if on the gingivae, can produce desquamative gingivitis — the most common oral finding. This is characterised by erythematous, ulcerated, tender gingivae in a patchy, rather than continuous distribution.

The majority of people with MMP have only oral lesions, but genital involvement can cause great morbidity and untreated ocular involvement can lead to blindness. Nasal, laryngeal and skin blisters are rare.

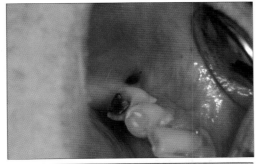

Fig. 3 Pemphigoid-showing blister

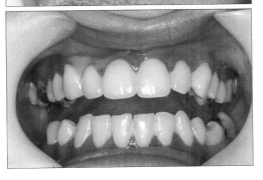

Fig. 4 Mucous membrane pemphigoid

Fig. 5 Pemphigoid: desquamative gingivitis

Diagnosis
The oral lesions of pemphigoid may be confused clinically with pemphigus, or occasionally erosive lichen planus, erythema multiforme or the sub-epithelial blistering conditions shown in Table 1.

Biopsy of perilesional tissue, with histological and immunostaining examination can therefore be essential to the diagnosis.

Management
Spontaneous remission is rare, and thus treatment is indicated. Specialist advice is usually needed.

Systemic manifestations must be given attention. For this reason, an ophthalmology consultation can be needed.

The majority of cases respond well to topical corticosteroids. Non-steroidal immunosuppressive agents such as tacrolimus may be needed if the response is inadequate.

Severe pemphigoid may need to be treated with immunosuppression using systemic azathioprine or corticosteroids.

Website and patient information
http://www.dent.ucla.edu/pic/members/MMP/index.html

PEMPHIGUS
Pemphigus is a group of fortunately rare, potentially life-threatening chronic diseases characterised by epithelial blistering affecting cutaneous and/or mucosal surfaces. There are several variants with different autoantibody profiles and clinical manifestations (Table 2) but the main type is pemphigus vulgaris; this includes an uncommon variant pemphigus vegetans. Pemphigus vulgaris is seen mainly in middle aged and elderly females of Mediterranean, Ashkenazi Jewish or South Asian descent.

Pemphigus vulgaris is an autoimmune disorder in which there is fairly strong genetic background. Rare cases have been triggered by medications (especially captopril, penicillamine, rifampicin and diclofenac) or other factors.

Table 2. Main types of pemphigus involving the mouth

Variant	Oral lesions	Main antigens	Localisation of antigens	Antibodies
Pemphigus vulgaris localised to mucosae (Mucosal)	Common	Dsg 3	Desmosomes	IgG
Pemphigus vulgaris also involving skin/ other mucosae (Muco-cutaneous)	Common	Dsg 3 Dsg 1	Desmosomes	IgG

The autoantibodies are directed against stratified squamous epithelial desmosomes, particularly the proteins desmoglein-3 (Dsg3) and plakoglobin (Table 2). Damage to the desmosomes leads to loss of cell-cell contact (acantholysis), and thus intra-epithelial vesiculation.

Clinical features
Pemphigus vulgaris typically runs a chronic course, causing blisters, erosions and ulcers on the mucosae and blisters and scabs on the skin. Oral lesions are common, may be an early manifestation and mimic those of pemphigoid in particular. Blisters rapidly break down to leave erosions seen mainly on the palate, buccal mucosa, lips and gingiva.

Diagnosis
To differentiate pemphigus from other vesiculobullous diseases, a careful history and physical examination are important, but biopsy of peri-lesional tissue, with histological and immunostaining examination are crucial. Serum should be collected for antibody titres.

Management
Before the introduction of corticosteroids, pemphigus vulgaris typically was fatal, mainly from dehydration or secondary systemic infections. Current treatment, by systemic immunosuppression, usually with steroids, or azathioprine or mycophenolate mofetil, has significantly reduced the mortality to about 10%. Specialist care is mandatory.

Websites and patient information
http://www.pemphigus.org

BLOOD DISORDERS
Blood disorders that can cause ulcers include mainly the leukaemias, associated with cytotoxic therapy, viral, bacterial or fungal infection, or non-specific. Other oral features of leukaemia may include purpura, gingival bleeding, recurrent herpes labialis, and candidosis.

Gastrointestinal disease may produce soreness or mouth ulcers. A few patients with aphthae have intestinal disease such as coeliac disease causing malabsorption and deficiencies of haematinics, when they may also develop angular stomatitis or glossitis. Crohn's disease and pyostomatitis vegetans may also cause ulcers. Orofacial granulomatosis (OFG), which has many features reminiscent of Crohn's disease, may also cause ulceration (see Chapter 8).

Other diseases such as lupus erythematosus can cause ulcers.

DIFFERENTIAL DIAGNOSIS OF ORAL ULCERATION
The most important feature of ulceration is whether the ulcer is single, multiple or persistent.

Multiple non-persistent ulcers are most commonly caused by viral infections or aphthae, when the ulcers heal spontaneously, usually within a week to a month. If this is not the case, or if the ulcers clinically do not appear to be aphthae, an alternative diagnosis should be considered.

A single ulcer that persists may be caused by neoplasia such as carcinoma or by chronic trauma, a chronic skin disease such as pemphigus, or a chronic infection such as syphilis, tuberculosis (TB) or a mycosis.

Multiple persistent ulcers are mainly caused by skin diseases such as lichen planus, pemphigoid or pemphigus, gastrointestinal disease, blood disease, immune defect or drugs.

In cases where the diagnosis is unclear, or where there is a single persistent ulcer, specialist referral is usually indicated.

DIAGNOSIS OF ORAL ULCERATION
Making a diagnosis of the cause for oral ulceration is based initially mainly on the history and clinical features. The number, persistence, shape, character of the edge of the ulcer and the appearance of the ulcer base should also be noted. Ulcers should always be examined for

induration (firmness on palpation), which may be indicative of malignancy. The cervical lymph nodes must be examined.

Unless the cause is undoubtedly local, general physical examination is also indicated, looking especially for mucocutaneous lesions, other lymphadenopathy or fever, since it is crucial to detect systemic causes such as leukaemia or HIV infection (Fig. 6).

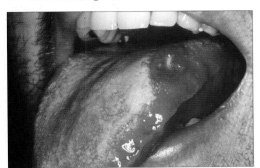

Fig. 6 HIV-associated ulceration

Investigations sometimes indicated include:
- blood tests to exclude haematinic deficiencies, leukaemia or HIV infection
- microbiological and serological investigations to exclude infection
- biopsy
- immunological studies to exclude skin diseases and HIV
- imaging to exclude TB, deep mycoses, carcinoma, or sarcoidosis.

Biopsy

Biopsy is indicated for persistent ulcers; where a dermatological casue is suspected; or where diagnosis is uncertain. Informed consent is mandatory for biopsy, particularly noting the likelihood of post-operative discomfort, and the possibility of bleeding or bruising or sensory loss. Care must be taken not to produce undue anxiety; some patients equate biopsy with a diagnosis of cancer. Perhaps the most difficult and important consideration is which part of the lesion should be included in the biopsy specimen.

As a general rule, the biopsy should include lesional and normal tissue. In the case of ulcerated mucosal lesions, most histopathological information is gleaned from the peri-lesional tissue since by definition most epithelium is lost from the ulcer itself. The same usually applies for skin diseases affecting the mouth, where the epithelium in the area mainly affected will, more often than not, separate before it ends up under the microscope, and results will be compromised. In the case of a suspected potentially malignant or malignant lesion, any red area should ideally be included in the specimen. In some cases where no obvious site can be chosen, vital staining with 'toluidine blue' may first be indicated (Chapter 9).

A biopsy punch has the advantage that the incision is controlled, an adequate specimen is obtained (typically 4 mm or 6 mm diameter) and suturing may not be required. However, in the skin disorders, the punch can sometimes split the epithelium or detach it from the lamina propria. When a scalpel is used, a specimen of elliptical shape is usually taken, most commonly from an edge of the lesion.

Procedure

A local analgesic should be given, although in a few cases, conscious sedation may also be necessary.

Make the incisions using a scalpel with a number 15 blade. Do not squeeze the specimen with forceps while trying to dissect the deep margin. A suture is best used for this purpose (and also to protect the specimen from going down the aspirator). Place the biopsy specimen on to a small piece of paper before immersing in fixative, to prevent curling.

Put the specimen into a labelled pot, ideally in at least 10 times its own volume of buffered formalin, and leave at room temperature.

Suture the wound if necessary, using resorbable sutures (eg Vicryl).

MANAGEMENT OF ORAL ULCERATION

- Treat the underlying cause
- Remove aetiological factors
- Prescribe a chlorhexidine 0.2% mouthwash
- Maintain good oral hygiene
- A benzydamine mouthwash or spray or other topical agents (Table 3) may help ease discomfort.

Table 3 Topical agents which may reduce pain from mucosal lesions

Agent	Use	Comments
Benzydamine hydrochloride	Rinse or spray every 1.5 to 3 hours	Effective in reducing discomfort
Lidocaine	Topical 4% solution may ease pain	Also reduces taste sensitivity
Carboxymethylcellulose	Paste or powder used after meals to protect area	Available containing triamcinolone May be religious objections to gelatin

REFERRAL OF PATIENTS WITH ORAL ULCERATION

Patients with single ulcers persisting more than three weeks, indurated ulcers, or multiple persistent ulcers may benefit from a specialist opinion.

Patients with recalcitrant ulcers, or a systemic background to mouth ulcers, or needing investigation, may also benefit from a specialist referral.

Features that might suggest a systemic background to mouth ulcers include:
- **Extraoral features** such as skin, ocular, or genital lesions (suggestive of Behçet's syndrome); purpura, fever, lymphadenopathy, hepatomegaly, or splenomegaly (which may be found in leukaemia), chronic cough (suggestive of TB or a mycosis), gastrointestinal complaints (eg pain, altered bowel habits, blood in faeces), weakness, loss of weight or, in children, a failure to thrive.
- **An atypical history or ulcer behaviour** such as onset of ulcers in later adult life, exacerbation of ulcers, severe aphthae, or aphthae unresponsive to topical steroids.
- **Other oral lesions**, especially infections suggestive of HIV/AIDS (candidosis, herpetic lesions, necrotising gingivitis or periodontitis, hairy leukoplakia or Kaposi's sarcoma) (Chapter 11), glossitis or angular cheilitis (suggestive of a haematinic state), or petechiae or gingival bleeding or swelling (raising the possibility of leukaemia).

Patients to refer

Malignancy
HIV related ulceration
Syphilis
TB
Drug related ulceration
Systemic disease
Mucocutaneous disorders

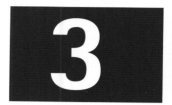
Dry mouth and disorders of salivation

Saliva is essential to oral health. The most obvious and important function of saliva is in eating, for taste and to lubricate food and protect the mucosa and teeth. The water, mucins and proline-rich glycoproteins lubricate food and help swallowing, and saliva is essential for normal taste perception. Saliva is protective via the washing action, via various antimicrobial components such as mucin, histatins, lysozyme and lactoferrin, and via specific antibodies to a range of micro-organisms that the host has encountered.

Salivary gland secretion from the major (parotid, submandibular and sublingual) and minor glands (multiple mucous glands scattered throughout the mouth — especially the lips and soft palate) is mainly under neural control, under the influence of the autonomic nervous system, although various hormones may also modulate its composition. In general, parasympathetic stimulation increases salivation, while sympathetic stimulation produces more viscous saliva and therefore appears to depress salivation.

Thus, in acute anxiety, when there is sympathetic stimulation, the mouth feels dry. The mouth is also dry if the parasympathetic system is inhibited by, for example, various drugs. Anything that damages the glands, or reduces body fluids can also reduce salivation.

DRY MOUTH (XEROSTOMIA)

Dry mouth (xerostomia) is a complaint that is the most common salivary problem and is the subjective sense of dryness which may be due to:

- Reduced salivary flow (hyposalivation) and/or
- Changed salivary composition.

Patients who have chronically decreased salivary flow (hyposalivation) suffer from lack of oral lubrication, affecting many functions, and they may complain of dryness (xerostomia), and can develop dental caries and other infections (candidosis, or acute bacterial sialadenitis) as a consequence of the reduced defences.

Causes

There are physiological causes of hyposalivation. Thus a dry mouth is common during periods of anxiety, due to sympathetic activity; mouthbreathers may also have a dry mouth and advancing age is associated with dry

Table 1 Causes of dry mouth
Iatrogenic
Drugs
Irradiation
Graft versus host disease
Disease
Dehydration (e.g. diabetes)
Psychogenic
Salivary gland disease
Sjögren's syndrome
Deposits (e.g. amyloid)
Sarcoidosis
Salivary aplasia
Infections (hepatitis C or HIV)

mouth - probably because of a reduction of salivary acini, with a fall in salivary secretory reserve.

Very rarely, children are born missing salivary glands — so-called salivary gland aplasia or agenesis. Most salivary gland dysfunction however is acquired (Table 1).

Drugs, in most older people complaining of xerostomia, are the cause. Indeed, the main causes of dry mouth are iatrogenic. There is usually a fairly close temporal relationship between starting the drug treatment or increasing the dose, and experiencing the dry mouth. However, the reason for which the drug is being taken may also be important. For example, patients with anxiety or depressive conditions may complain of dry mouth even in the absence of drug therapy (or evidence of reduced salivary flow).

Drugs recognised as causes of reduced salivation include mainly those with anticholinergic, or sympathomimetic, or diuretic activity. These include those shown in Table 2 and Chapter 11.

Irradiation for malignant tumours in the head and neck region, such as oral cancer, can produce profound xerostomia. Other sources of irradiation such as radioactive iodine (^{131}I) used for treating thyroid disease, may also damage the salivary glands, which take up the radioactive iodine. Graft versus host disease may cause xerostomia.

Dehydration, as in diabetes mellitus, chronic renal failure, hyperparathyroidism, any fever or diabetes insipidus can cause xerostomia.

Diseases of salivary glands can also cause salivary dysfunction. These are mainly Sjögren's syndrome (a multisystem auto-immune condition discussed below); sarcoidosis; HIV disease; hepatitis C virus infection; liver diseases; cystic fibrosis (mucoviscidosis) and various deposits in the glands (Fig. 1).

Finally, it is important to also recognise that some patients complaining of a dry mouth have no evidence of a reduced salivary flow or a salivary disorder (ie they have xerostomia but not hyposalivation), and in these there may be a psychogenic reason for the complaint.

Clinical features

The patient with hyposalivation may have difficulty in:
- Swallowing — especially dry foods such as biscuits (the cracker sign)
- Controlling dentures
- Speaking, as the tongue tends to stick to the palate — leading to 'clicking' speech.

Patients may also complain of unpleasant taste or loss of sense of taste, or halitosis.

The patient with hyposalivation may complain of a dry mouth or these sequelae alone, or also complain of dryness of the eyes and other mucosae (nasal, laryngeal, genital). Those with eye complaints may have blurring, light intolerance, burning, itching or grittiness, and sometimes an inability to cry.

Systemic features (such as joint pains) may be suggestive of Sjögren's syndrome.

Examination may reveal that the lips adhere one to another and an examining dental mirror may stick to the mucosa because of the reduced lubrication. Lipstick or food debris may be seen sticking to the teeth or soft tissues, and the usual pooling of saliva in the floor of the mouth may be absent. Thin lines of frothy saliva may form along lines of contact of the oral soft tissues, on the tongue, or in the vestibule. Saliva may not be expressible from the parotid ducts. The tongue is dry (Fig. 2) and may become lobulated and usually red, with partial or complete depapillation (Fig. 3).

Complications of hyposalivation can include:
- Dental caries — which tends to involve smooth surfaces and areas otherwise not very prone to caries — such as the lower incisor region and roots. Hyposalivation may

Table 2 Drugs associated with dry mouth
Drugs which directly damage the salivary glands
Cytotoxic drugs
Drugs with anticholinergic activity
Anticholinergic agents such as atropine, atropinics and hyoscine
Antireflux agents eg proton-pump inhibitors (such as omeprazole)
Psychoactive agents with anticholinergic activities such as:
Antidepressants, including tricyclic (eg amitriptyline, nortriptyline, clomipramine and dothiepin [dosulepin]), selective serotonin re-uptake inhibitors (eg fluoxetine), lithium and others.
Phenothiazines
Benzodiazepines
Opioids
Antihistamines
Bupropion
Drugs acting on sympathetic system
Drugs with sympathomimetic activity eg ephedrine
Antihypertensives; alpha 1 antagonists (e.g. terazosin and prazosin) and alpha 2 agonists (e.g. clonidine) may reduce salivary flow. Beta blockers (e.g. atenolol, propranolol) also change salivary protein levels.
Drugs which deplete fluid
Diuretics

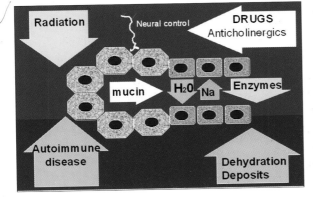

Fig. 1 Saliva production and factors inhibiting it (arrowed)

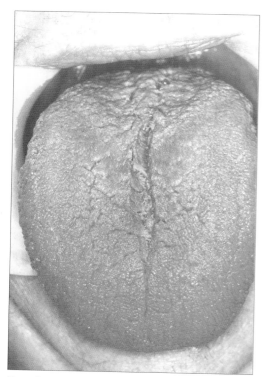

Fig. 2 Dry mouth

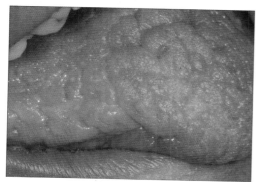

Fig. 3 Dry mouth and lobulated tongue

explain patients with uncontrollable recurrent caries, who are apparently complying with dietary advice.

- Candidosis (Fig. 4) – which may cause a burning sensation or mucosal erythema, lingual filiform papillae atrophy, and angular stomatitis (angular cheilitis)
- Halitosis (Chapter 4)
- Ascending (suppurative) sialadenitis – which

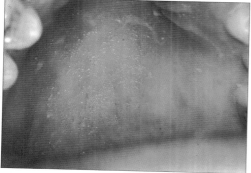

Fig. 4 Dry mouth complicated by candidosis

presents with pain and swelling of a major salivary gland, and sometimes purulent discharge from the duct.

Diagnosis

Hyposalivation is a clinical diagnosis which can be made by the practitioner predominantly on the basis of the history and examination.

It can be helpful to document salivary function by salivary function studies such as salivary flow rates (sialometry). Collection of whole saliva (oral fluid) is currently the routine technique for sialometry used by many clinicians, despite the fact that it is rather inaccurate and non-specific. It is usually carried out by allowing the patient to sit quietly and dribble into a measuring container over 15 minutes; in a normal person, such an unstimulated whole saliva flow rate exceeds 1.5 ml/15 min (0.1 ml/min).

The specialist may be needed to:
- Study and document the degree of salivary dysfunction
- Determine the cause
- Arrange future dental care although much of this can be undertaken in the primary care environment.

Investigations may be indicated to exclude systemic disease, particularly to exclude:
- Sjögren's syndrome and connective tissue disorders
- Diabetes
- Sarcoidosis
- Viral infections (hepatitis C; HIV).

Commonly used investigations may thus include:
- Blood tests (mainly to exclude diabetes, Sjögren's syndrome, sarcoidosis, hepatitis and other infections)
- Eye tests (eg Schirmer test mainly to exclude Sjögren's syndrome)
- Salivary gland biopsy (if there is suspicion of organic disease such as Sjögren's syndrome)
- Imaging (mainly to exclude Sjögren's syndrome, sarcoidosis or neoplasia).

It is important to remember, as stated above, that in some patients complaining of a dry mouth no evidence of a reduced salivary flow or a salivary disorder can be found. There may then be a psychogenic reason for the complaint.

Management (see below)

SJÖGREN'S SYNDROME

Sjögren's syndrome (SS) is an uncommon condition, the association of dry mouth and dry eyes. The other key features of SS are evidence of an autoimmune reaction shown usually by serum autoantibodies and sometimes confirmed by demonstrating mononuclear cell infiltrates in a labial salivary gland biopsy. Sjögren's syndrome can affect any age but the onset is most common in middle age or older. The majority of patients are women.

Aetiopathogenesis

SS is an autoimmune disease affecting mainly exocrine glands like the salivary glands, lacrimal glands and pancreas. There may be a viral aetiology and a genetic predisposition.

The most common type of SS is secondary Sjögren's syndrome (SS-2) which comprises dry eyes and dry mouth and a connective tissue or autoimmune disease usually rheumatoid arthritis (RA) (Table 3). However, SS can appear by itself and, in the absence of a connective tissue disease is often termed sicca syndrome, usually referred to as primary Sjögren's syndrome (SS-1). Nevertheless, both forms are chronic and can affect not only the salivary glands (Fig. 5), but also extraglandular tissues. Chronic B lymphocyte stimulation can occasionally lead to B cell neoplasms such as lymphoma.

Table 3 Sjögren's syndrome

	SS-1	SS-2
Dry mouth	Yes	Yes
Dry eyes	Yes	Yes
Connective tissue disease	No	Yes
Extraglandular problems	More common	Less common

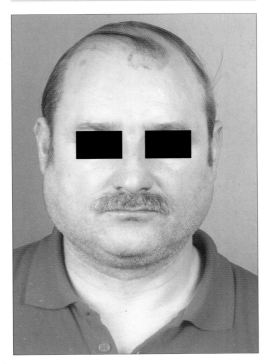

Fig. 5 Parotid gland swelling

SS is often characterised by a raised erythrocyte sedimentation rate (ESR) and several autoantibodies — particularly antinuclear factor (ANF) and rheumatoid factor (RF), and more specific antinuclear antibodies known as SS-A (Ro) and SS-B (La).

Clinical features

SS presents mainly with eye complaints which include sensations of grittiness, soreness, itching, dryness, blurred vision or light intolerance. The eyes may be red with inflammation of the conjunctivae and soft crusts at the angles (keratoconjunctivitis sicca). The lacrimal glands may swell.

Oral complaints (often the presenting feature) including:
- Xerostomia
- Swollen salivary glands; causes include chronic sialadenitis as part of the fundamental autoimmune disease process, ascending bacterial sialadenitis which can arise if bacteria ascend the ducts because salivation is

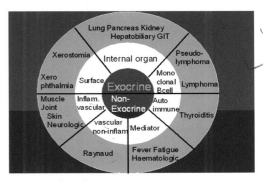

Fig. 6 Complications of Sjögren's syndrome

impaired, benign lymphoepithelial lesions/ myoepithelial sialadenitis (pseudolymphoma) and lymphoma (Fig. 6).

However, SS is a more generalised disorder which involves not only the exocrine salivary and lacrimal glands, but can have a range of other complications, summarised in Figure 6.

Diagnosis

Diagnosis is made from the history and clinical features, and may be confirmed by autoantibody studies and sometimes by other investigations such as sialometry imaging and labial salivary gland biopsy. In specialist units various international criteria are used to confirm the diagnosis. There is no specific treatment yet for SS, but the hyposalivation can be managed, and dental preventive care is essential. The dental team have an important role to play in this.

Management of hyposalivation

Any underlying cause of xerostomia should if possible be rectified; for example, xerostomia-producing drugs may be changed for an alternative, and causes such as diabetes should be treated.

Patients should be educated into efforts to avoid factors that may increase dryness , and to keep the mouth moist (Table 4).

Salivary substitutes may help symptomatically. A variety are available including:
- Water or ice chips; frequent sips of water are generally effective
- Synthetic salivary substitutes (Table 5).

As patients with objective xerostomia are at increased risk of developing caries it is important that they take a non-cariogenic diet and maintain a high standard of oral hygiene. The regular use of topical fluoride agents forms an

Table 4 Ten tips for managing a dry mouth

1 Drink enough water, and sip on water and other non-sugary fluids throughout the day. Rinse with water after meals. Keep water at your bedside.

2 Replace missing saliva with salivary substitutes, eg Artificial Saliva, (Glandosane, Luborant, Biotene Oralbalance, AS Saliva Orthana, Salivace, Saliveze). Alcohol-free mouthrinses (BioXtra and Biotène), or moisturising gels (Oralbalance, BioXtra) may help.

3 Stimulate saliva with:
   - sugar-free chewing gums (eg EnDeKay, Orbit, Biotène dry mouth gum or BioXtra chewing gum) or
   - diabetic sweets or
   - Salivix or SST if advised or
   - drugs that stimulate salivation (eg pilocarpine [Salagen]) if advised by a specialist.

4 Always take water or non-alcoholic drinks with meals

5 Avoid dry or hard crunchy foods such as biscuits, or dunk in liquids. Take small bites and eat slowly. Eat soft creamy foods (casseroles, soups), or cool foods with a high liquid content — melon, grapes, or ice cream. Moisten foods with gravies, sauces, extra oil, margarine, salad dressings, sour cream, mayonnaise or yogurt. Pineapple has an enzyme that helps clean the mouth. Avoid spices.

6 Avoid anything that may worsen dryness, such as:
   - drugs, unless they are essential (eg antidepressants)
   - alcohol (including in mouthwashes)
   - smoking
   - caffeine (coffee, some soft drinks such as colas)
   - mouthbreathing.

7 Protect against dental caries by avoiding sugary foods/drinks and by:
   - reducing sugar intake (avoid snacking and eating last thing at night)
   - avoiding sticky foods such as toffee
   - keeping your mouth very clean (twice daily toothbrushing and flossing)
   - using a fluoride toothpaste
   - using fluoride gels or mouthwashes (0.05% fluoride) daily before going to bed
   - having regular dental checks.

8 Protect against thrush, gum problems and halitosis by:
   - keeping your mouth very clean
   - keeping your mouth as moist as possible
   - rinsing twice daily with chlorhexidine (eg Chlorohex, Corsodyl, Eludril) or triclosan (eg Plax)
   - brushing or scraping your tongue
   - keeping dentures out at night
   - disinfecting dentures in hypochlorite (eg Milton, Dentural)
   - using antifungals if recommended by specialist.

9 Protect the lips with a lip salve or petroleum jelly (eg Vaseline).

10 Avoid hot, dry environments — consider a humidifier for the bedroom.

Table 5 Some salivary replacements

UK trade names	Offered as	Contains fluoride	Main constituents	Comments
AS Saliva Orthana	Spray or lozenge	+ /-	Mucin Xylitol	Spray contains fluoride but is unsuitable if there are religious objections to porcine mucin
Biotene Oralbalance	Gel	-	Glycerate polymer base, lactoperoxidase, glucose oxidase, xylitol	
BioXtra	Gel	-	Colostrum, lactoperoxidase, glucose oxidase, xylitol	
Luborant	Spray	+	Carboxymethylcellulose	May contain fluoride
Glandosane	Spray	-	Carboxymethylcellulose	Low pH
Salivace	Spray		Carboxymethylcellulose	
Saliveze	Spray		Carboxymethylcellulose	

Useful websites:
- http://www.arc.org.uk/about_arth/booklets/6041/6041.htm
- http://www.nidcr.nih.gov/HealthInformation/DiseasesAndConditions/SjogrensSyndrome.htm
- http://www.sjsworld.org/
- http://www.nidcr.nih.gov/HealthInformation/DiseasesAndConditions/DryMouthXerostomia/drymouth.htm
- http://www.oralcancerfoundation.org/dental/xerostomia.htm

SIALORRHOEA (HYPERSALIVATION; PTYALISM)

Infants frequently drool but this is normal. The complaint of sialorrhoea (excess salivation) is uncommon and may be true salivary hypersecretion — usually caused by physiological factors such as menstruation or early pregnancy, local factors such as teething or oral inflammatory lesions, food or medications (those with cholinergic activity such as pilocarpine, tetrabenazine, clozapine), or by nasogastric intubation. In some cases, apparent hypersalivation is caused not by excess saliva production but by an inability to swallow a normal amount of saliva (false sialorrhoea) caused by neuromuscular dysfunction (eg in Parkinson's disease, cerebral palsy, or learning disability) or by pharyngeal or oesophageal obstruction, such as by a neoplasm.

Treatment is of the underlying cause if possible and then the use of behavioural approaches or antisialogogues. Occasionally, surgery to redirect the salivary gland ducts into the oropharynx may be helpful.

important component of their long-term care.

Salivation may be stimulated by using diabetic sweets or chewing gums (containing sorbitol or xylitol, not sucrose). Cholinergic drugs that stimulate salivation (sialogogues), such as pilocarpine, or cevimeline should be used only by a specialist. Oral complications should be prevented and treated.

Patients to refer
Suspected Sjögren's syndrome

Oral malodour

ORAL MALODOUR

Oral malodour, or halitosis, is a common complaint in adults, though few mention it. Malodour can have a range of causes (Table 1). With oral malodour from any cause, the patient may also complain of a bad taste.

Table 1 Main causes of oral malodour

Oral sepsis
Dry mouth
Starvation
Some foods
Habits: smoking, alcohol and some drugs
Systemic disease
Diabetic ketosis
Gastrointestinal disease
Hepatic failure
Renal failure
Respiratory disease
Trimethylaminuria
Psychogenic factors

Common causes of oral malodour

Oral malodour is common on awakening (morning breath) and then often has no special significance — usually being a consequence of low salivary flow and lack of oral cleansing during sleep as well as mouthbreathing.

This can be readily rectified by eating, tongue brushing, and rinsing the mouth with fresh water. Hydrogen peroxide rinses may also help abolish this odour.

Oral malodour at other times is often the consequence of eating various foods such as garlic, onion or spices, foods such as cabbage, Brussel sprouts, cauliflower and radish, or of habits such as smoking, or drinking alcohol. Durian is a tropical fruit which is particularly malodourous.

The cause of malodour in such cases is usually obvious and avoidance of the offending substance is the best prevention.

Less common causes of oral malodour

Oral infections can be responsible for oral malodour. The micro—organisms implicated in oral malodour are predominantly Gram-negative anaerobes, and include:
- *Porphyromonas gingivalis*
- *Prevotella intermedia*
- *Fusobacterium nucleatum*
- *Bacteroides (Tannerella) forsythensis* and
- *Treponema denticola.*

Gram-positive bacteria have also been implicated since they can denude the available glycoproteins of their sugar chains, enabling the anaerobic Gram-negative proteolytic bacteria to break down the proteins. Gram-negative bacteria can produce chemicals that produce malodour, which include in many instances
- volatile sulphur compounds (VSCs), mainly methyl mercaptan, hydrogen sulphide, and dimethyl sulphide
- diamines (putrescine and cadaverine) and
- short chain fatty acids (butyric, valeric and propionic).

The evidence for the implication of other micro-organisms, such as *Helicobacter pylori*, is scant.

The posterior area of the tongue dorsum is often the location of the microbial activity associated with bad breath. Plaque and debris, such as in patients with poor oral hygiene, or under a neglected or a poorly designed dental bridge or appliance is another cause. Any patient with oral cancer or a dry mouth can also develop oral malodour.

Defined infective processes that can cause malodour may include:

- Periodontal infections (especially necrotising gingivitis or periodontitis)
- Pericoronitis
- Other types of oral infections
- Infected extraction sockets
- Ulcers.

Improvement of oral hygiene, prevention or treatment of infective processes, and sometimes the use of antimicrobials can usually manage this type of oral malodour.

Rare causes of oral malodour

Systemic causes of oral malodour are rare but important and range from drugs to sepsis in the respiratory tract to metabolic disorders (Table 2).

The complaint of oral malodour in the absence of malodour

The complaint of oral malodour may be made by patients who do not have it but imagine it because of psychogenic reasons. This can be a real clinical dilemma, since no evidence of oral malodour can be detected even with objective testing, and the oral malodour may then be attributable to a form of delusion or monosymptomatic hypochondriasis (self-oral malodour; halitophobia).

Other people's behaviour, or perceived behaviour, such as apparently covering the nose or averting the face, is typically misinterpreted by these patients as an indication that their breath is indeed offensive. Such patients may have latent psychosomatic illness tendencies.

Many of these patients will adopt behaviour to minimise their perceived problem, such as

- covering the mouth when talking
- avoiding or keeping a distance from other people
- avoiding social situations
- using chewing gum, mints, mouthwashes or sprays designed to reduce malodour
- frequent toothbrushing
- cleaning their tongue.

Thus the oral hygiene may be superb in such patients. Medical help may be required to manage these patients.

Such patients unfortunately fail to recognise their own psychological condition, never doubt they have oral malodour and thus are often reluctant to visit a psychologic specialist.

Summary

Oral malodour can have a range of causes, though most cases of true malodour have an oral cause, and many others are imagined (Fig. 1).

DIAGNOSIS OF ORAL MALODOUR

Assessment of oral malodour is usually subjective by simply smelling exhaled air (organoleptic method) coming from the mouth and nose and comparing the two. Odour originating in the mouth, but not detectable from the nose is likely to be either oral or pharyngeal origin. Odour originating in the nose may come from the sinuses or nasal passages. Children sometimes place foreign bodies in the nose, leading to sepsis and malodour! Only in the rare cases in which similar odour is equally sensed coming from both the nose and mouth can one of the many systemic causes be inferred.

Specialist centres may have the apparatus for objectively measuring the responsible volatile sulphur compounds (methyl mercaptan, hydrogen sulphide, dimethyl sulphide) – a halimeter. Microbiological investigations such as the BANA (benzoyl-arginine-naphthylamide) test or darkfield microscopy can also be helpful.

Management of oral malodour

The management includes first determining which cases may have an extraoral aetiology.

A full oral examination is indicated and if an oral cause is likely or possible, management should include treatment of the cause, and other measures (see box).

In cases of malodour which may have an extraoral aetiology, the responsibility of the general dental practitioner is to refer the patient for

Table 2. Rare causes of oral malodour

Drugs
  Chloral hydrate
  Cytotoxic drugs
  Dimethyl sulphoxide
  Nitrites and nitrates
  Solvent abuse
Respiratory problems
  Nasal sepsis
  Tonsillitis
  Sinusitis
  Lower respiratory tract infection
Systemic disease
  Diabetic ketosis; the breath may smell of acetone
  Gastrointestinal disease: (some believe in an association with Helicobacter pylori infection)
  Hepatic failure
  Renal failure.
  Trimethylaminuria (fish-malodour syndrome); an autosomal dominant metabolic disorder. Trimethylamine (TMA) is produced by intestinal bacteria on eating cholines (mainly in fish and eggs) and is typically oxidised by a liver enzyme. Individuals with trimethylaminuria lack this enzyme and thus secrete TMA in various bodily fluids and via their breath.
  Psychogenic factors

Keypoints for dentists: Malodour (Halitosis)

- Malodour is common on awakening (morning breath)
- If real is usually caused by diet, habits, dental plaque or oral disease
- It can be measured with a halimeter
- It often significantly improves with oral hygiene
- It can sometimes be caused by sinus, nose or throat conditions
- It is rarely caused by more serious disease

Key points for patients: 11 steps towards control of oral malodour

- Treat any identifiable cause (this may need antimicrobials)
- Avoid odiferous foods such as onions, garlic, spices and durian
- Avoid habits that may worsen breath odour, such as;

    alcohol

    tobacco

- Eat a good breakfast, and take regular meals including fresh fruit: an enzyme in pineapple (papain) helps clean the mouth
- Brush your teeth after meals
- Keep oral hygiene regular and good

    Prophylaxis

    Toothbrushing

    Flossing

- Rinse at least twice daily with chlorhexidine (eg Chlorohex, Corsodyl, Eludril), triclosan (Total), essential oils (Listerine), cetylpyridinium (MacLeans), chlorine dioxide (Retardex) or other mouthwashes
- Brush your tongue before going to bed: use a tongue scraper if that helps
- Keep your mouth as moist as possible by using

    sugar-free chewing gums (eg Orbit, EnDeKay)

    diabetic sweets

- Use proprietary 'fresh breath' preparations eg Dentyl pH
- If you have dentures, leave them out at night and in hypochlorite (eg Dentural) or chlorhexidine.

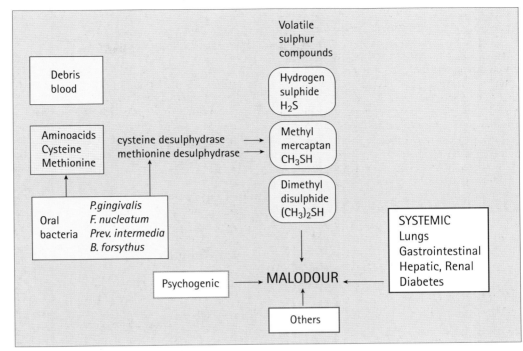

Fig. 1 Causes of malodour

evaluation to a specialist. This may involve an oral medicine opinion, an otorhinolaryngologist to rule out the presence of chronic tonsillitis or chronic sinusitis, a physician to rule out gastric, hepatic, endocrine, pulmonary, metabolic or renal disease or a psychologist or psychiatrist.

Patient information and websites
http://www.tau.ac.il/~melros/

Patients to refer
Suspected systemic disease
Suspected malignancy

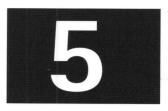

IN BRIEF
- Most white lesions in the mouth are inconsequential and caused by friction or trauma.
- However, cancer, potentially malignant diseases and some systemic diseases such as lichen planus and candidosis may present in this way.
- Biopsy may be indicated.

Oral white patches

WHITE LESIONS

Truly white oral lesions may consist of collections of debris (materia alba), or necrotic epithelium (such as after a burn), or fungi – such as candidosis. These can typically be wiped off the mucosa with a gauze.

Other lesions which cannot be wiped off, appear white usually because they are composed of thickened keratin, which looks white when wet (Fig. 1). A few rare conditions that are congenital, such as white sponge naevus (Fig. 2) present in this way but most such white lesions are acquired and many were formerly known as 'leukoplakia', a term causing misunderstanding and confusion. The World Health Organisation originally defined leukoplakia as a 'white patch or plaque that cannot be characterised clinically or pathologically as any other disease', therefore specifically excluding defined clinicopathologic entities such as can-

didosis, lichen planus (LP) and white sponge naevus, but still incorporating white lesions caused by friction or other trauma, and offering no comment on the presence of dysplasia. A subsequent seminar defined leukoplakia more precisely, as 'a whitish patch or plaque that cannot be characterised clinically or pathologically as any other disease and which is not associated with any physical or chemical causative agent except the use of tobacco'.

There are a range of causes of white lesions (Table 1). Morphological features may give a guide to the diagnosis. For example, focal lesions are often caused by keratoses. Multifocal lesions are common in thrush (pseudomembranous candidosis) and in LP. Striated lesions are typical of LP, and diffuse white areas are seen in the buccal mucosa in leukoedema and some LP, in the palate in stomatitis nicotina and at any site in keratoses. White lesions are usually pain-

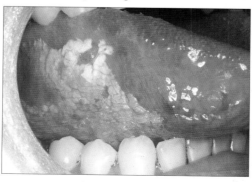

Fig. 1 Leukoplakia, ventral tongue

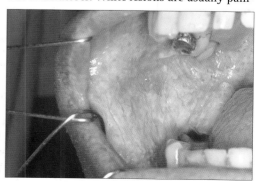

Fig. 2 White sponge naevus

Table 1 Causes of oral white lesions

Local causes
- Materia alba and furred tongue (debris from poor oral hygiene)
- Burns
- Keratoses
    - Frictional keratosis (and cheek/lip biting)
    - Smoker's keratosis
    - Snuff-dipper's keratosis
- Skin grafts
- Scars

Congenital
- Fordyce spots
- Leukoedema
- Inherited dyskeratoses (rare eg white sponge naevus, dyskeratosis congenita, Darier's disease)

Inflammatory
    Infective
- Fungal (eg candidosis)
- Viral
    - Hairy leukoplakia (Epstein-Barr virus)
    - Human papillomavirus infections
- Bacterial (eg syphilitic mucous patches and keratosis)

    Non-infective
- Lichen planus
- Lupus erythematosus

Neoplastic and possibly pre-neoplastic
- Leukoplakia
- Keratoses
- Carcinoma

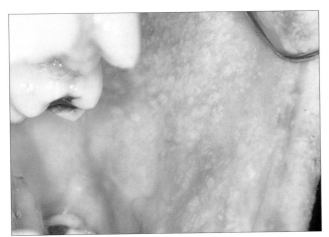

Fig. 3 Fordyce spots

less but this may not be the case in burns, candidosis, LP, or lupus erythematosus.

Local causes of white lesions

Debris, burns (from heat, radiation, chemicals such as mouthwashes), grafts and scars may appear pale or white. Materia alba can usually easily be wiped off with a gauze.

Furred tongue

Tongue coating is common, particularly in edentulous adults on a soft, non-abrasive diet, people with poor oral hygiene, and those who are fasting or have febrile diseases. The coating appears more obvious in xerostomia. The coating may be white, yellow or brown and consists of epithelial, food and microbial debris and the tongue is the main reservoir of some micro-organisms such as *Candida albicans* and some *Streptococci*, and the various anaerobes implicated in oral malodour (see Chapter 4).

Diagnosis

The history is important to exclude a congenital or hereditary cause of a white lesion. The clinical appearances usually strongly suggest the diagnosis. Biopsy is only required if the white lesion cannot be rubbed off from the mucosa with a gauze.

Management

Treatment is of the underlying cause where this can be identified.

CONGENITAL CAUSES OF WHITE LESIONS

Fordyce spots

Some common whitish conditions, notably Fordyce granules (ectopic sebaceous glands) are really yellowish, but may cause diagnostic confusion (Fig. 3). This condition is entirely benign and does not require any further intervention.

Leukoedema

Leukoedema is a common benign congenital whitish-grey filmy appearance of the mucosa, seen especially in the buccal mucosae bilaterally in persons of African or Asian descent. Diagnosis is clinical – the white appearance disappears if the mucosa is stretched. No treatment is available or required.

Inherited dyskeratoses

Inherited disorders of keratin are rare, but may be diagnosed from a family history or other features associated, such as lesions on other mucosae, or skin appendages such as the nails.

White sponge naevus, the commonest of the inherited dyskeratoses, is an autosomal dominant condition characterised by thickened, folded white patches most commonly affecting the buccal mucosae (Fig. 2). Other mucosal sites in the mouth may be involved and some patients may have similar lesions affecting genital and rectal mucosa.

Since other dyskeratoses may have wider implications and in particular the risk of malignant transformation, specialist care is indicated.

INFLAMMATORY CAUSES OF WHITE LESIONS

Infections

White lesions which can result from infections include candidosis (Fig. 4), hairy leukoplakia (caused by Epstein-Barr virus), warts and papillomas (caused by human papillomaviruses) (Fig. 5) and the mucous patches and leukoplakia of syphilis. Specialist care is usually indicated.

Candidosis (candidiasis; moniliasis)

The importance of *Candida* has increased greatly, particularly as the HIV pandemic extends. This

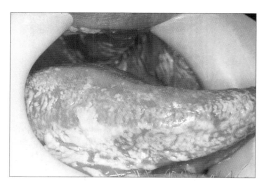

Fig. 4 Pseudomembranous candidosis

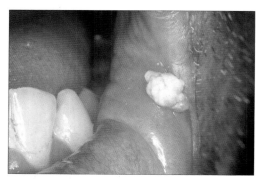

Fig. 5 Condyloma acuminatum (genital wart)

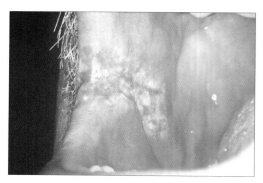

Fig. 6 Candidal leukoplakia, right buccal mucosa

common commensal can become opportunistic if local ecology changes, or the host immune defences fail. *Candida albicans* is the common cause but occasionally other species may be implicated; in decreasing order of frequency these are:

- *C. tropicalis*
- *C. glabrata*
- *C. parapsilosis*
- *C. krusei*
- Other *Candida* species and other genera.

Some 50% of the normal healthy population harbour (carry) *C. albicans* as a normal oral commensal particularly on the posterior dorsum of tongue, and are termed *Candida* carriers.

Candidosis is the state when *C. albicans* causes lesions and these can be mainly white lesions; (thrush particularly; Fig. 4) or candidal leukoplakia (Fig. 6) in which hyphal forms are common, or red lesions (denture-related stomatitis, median rhomboid glossitis, erythematous candidosis) — in which yeast forms predomi-

nate, and which may be symptomless though antibiotic stomatitis and angular cheilitis can cause soreness (Chapter 6).

Circumstances that cause susceptibility to candidosis include local factors influencing oral immunity or ecology, or systemic immune defects, or a combination of more than one factor (Table 2).

Diagnosis

The diagnosis of candidosis is clinical usually but a Gram-stained smear (hyphae) or oral rinse may help.

Management

Possible predisposing causes should be looked for and dealt with, if possible. Polyene antifungals such as nystatin or amphotericin, or imidazoles such as miconazole or fluconazole are often indicated.

Non-infective causes

Lichen planus (LP) is a very common cause of oral white lesions. Most dental practitioners will have patients afflicted with LP. It is the main skin disease that can present with oral white lesions but lupus erythematosus and keratoses can present similarly.

Lichen planus

Lichen planus (LP) usually affects persons between the ages of 30 to 65 and there is a slight female predisposition.

Aetiopathogenesis

LP is an inflammatory autoimmune type of disease but it differs from classic autoimmune disorders in having no defined autoantibodies, and only rarely being associated with other autoimmune diseases. There is also no definitive immunogenetic basis yet established for LP and familial cases are rare.

Many patients afflicted with LP have a conscientious type of personality with obsessive-compulsive traits and suffer mild chronic anxiety, suggesting neuro-immunological mechanisms may be at play. Stress has been held to be important in LP: patients have a tendency to be anxious and depressed, but of course the chronic discomfort may partially explain some cases in which this association has been documented.

Pathologically, there is a local cell-mediated immunological response characterised by a

Table 2 Factors predisposing to candidosis

Local factors influencing oral immunity or ecology	Systemic immune defects
Xerostomia	Malnutrition
Smoking	Immunosuppressant drugs such as corticosteroids
Corticosteroids	T lymphocyte defects, especially HIV infection, leukaemias, lymphomas, and cancers
Broad spectrum antimicrobials	Neutrophil leukocyte defects, such as in diabetes
Cytotoxic chemotherapy	Cytotoxic chemotherapy
Irradiation involving the mouth/salivary glands	Anaemia
Dental appliances	

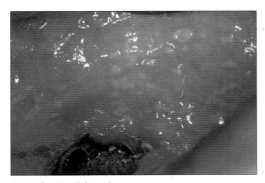

Fig. 7 Papular lichen planus

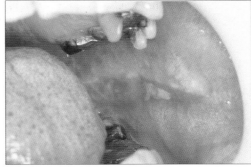

Fig. 10 Erosive and atrophic lichen planus, buccal mucosa

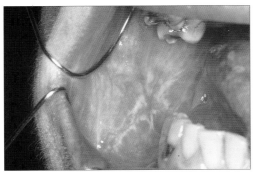

Fig. 8 Reticular lichen planus

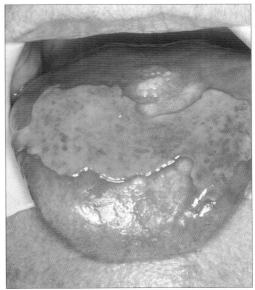

Fig. 11 Erosive lichen planus, dorsum of tongue

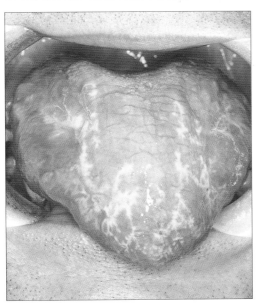

Fig. 9 Reticular lichen planus, dorsum of tongue

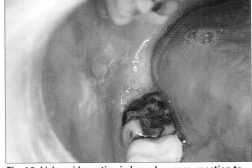

Fig. 12 Lichenoid reaction in buccal mucosa, reaction to amalgam contact

dense T lymphocyte inflammatory cell infiltrate in the upper lamina propria causing cell death (apoptosis) in the basal epithelium, probably caused by the production of cytokines such as tumour-necrosis factor alpha (TNF-α) and interferon gamma (IFN-γ).

The antigen responsible for this immune response is unclear but lesions very similar to LP – termed lichenoid lesions – are sometimes caused by:

- Dental restorative materials (mainly amalgam and gold)
- Drugs (non- steroidal anti-inflammatory agents, antihypertensive agents antimalarials, and many other drugs)

- Chronic graft-versus-host disease seen in bone marrow (haemopoietic stem cell) transplant patients
- Infection with hepatitis C virus (HCV) in some populations such as those from southern Europe and Japan
- A variety of other systemic disorders such as hypertension and diabetes – probably a reaction to the drugs used.

Clinical features

LP can affect stratified squamous epithelium of the skin, the oral mucosa and genitalia.

Oral LP may present a number of different clinical pictures (Figs 7–12), including:

- Papular LP – white papules (Fig. 7)
- Reticular LP – a network of raised white lines or striae (reticular pattern) (Figs 8 and 9)
- Plaque-like LP – simulating leukoplakia
- Atrophic red atrophic areas – simulating erythroplasia (Fig. 10; mixed atrophic/erosive form): lichen planus is one of the most common cause of desquamative gingivitis.
- Erosive erosions – less common, but persistent, irregular, and painful, with a yellowish slough (Fig. 11).

White lesions of LP are often asymptomatic, but there may be soreness if there are atrophic areas or erosions.

LP typically results in lesions in the posterior buccal mucosa bilaterally but the tongue or gingivae are other sites commonly affected.

On the skin, lichen planus frequently presents as a flat-topped purple polygonal and pruritic papular rash most often seen on the front (flexor surface) of the wrists (Fig. 13) in which lesions are often are crossed by fine white lines (Wickham's striae; Fig. 14). Oral LP may be accompanied by vulvovaginal lesions (the vulvovaginal-gingival syndrome) or penile lesions.

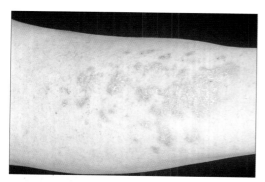

Fig. 13 Lichen planus, skin

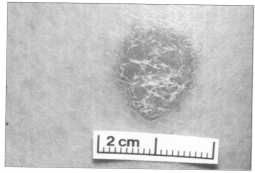

Fig. 14 Cutaneous lichen planus

Prognosis

Often the onset of LP is slow, taking months to reach its peak. It may clear from the skin within 18 months but in a few people persists for many years. Oral lesions often persist. There is no sign or test to indicate which patients will develop only oral, or oral and extraoral lesions of LP.

Non-reticular oral LP in particular has a small premalignant potential – probably of the order of 1%. There is no test to reliably predict this.

Diagnosis

LP is often fairly obviously diagnosed from the clinical features but, since it can closely simulate other conditions such as:

- Lupus erythematosus,
- Chronic ulcerative stomatitis,
- Keratosis, or even
- Carcinoma,

biopsy and histopathological examination of lesional tissue, occasionally aided by direct immunostaining, are often indicated.

Management

Treatment of LP is not always necessary, unless there are symptoms. Predisposing factors should be corrected:

- It may be wise to consider removal of dental amalgams if the lesions are closely related to these, or unilateral, but tests such as patch tests will not reliably indicate which patients will benefit from this. Accordingly, empirical replacement of amalgam restorations may be indicated.
- If drugs are implicated, the physician should be consulted as to the possibility of changing drug therapy.
- If there is HCV infection, this should be managed by a general physician.
- Improvement in oral hygiene may result in some subjective benefit; chlorhexidine or triclosan mouthwashes may help. Symptoms can often be controlled, usually with topical corticosteroids or sometimes with tacrolimus.
- If there is severe or extensive oral involvement, if LP fails to respond to topical medications, or if there are extraoral lesions, specialist referral may be indicated.
- Patients with non-reticular lichen planus should be monitored to exclude development of carcinoma. Tobacco and alcohol use should be minimised.

Changes that might suggest a tumour is developing could include any of the following persisting more than three weeks:

- An ulcer on the lip or in the mouth that does not heal
- A lump on the lip or in the mouth or throat
- A white or red lesion on the gums, tongue, or lining of the mouth
- Unusual bleeding, pain, or numbness in the mouth
- A sore throat that does not go away, or a feeling that something is caught in the throat
- Difficulty or pain with chewing or swallowing
- Swelling of the jaw that causes dentures to fit poorly or become uncomfortable
- Pain in the ear
- Enlargement of a neck lymph gland.

Websites and patient information
http://www.tambcd.edu/lichen/
http://www.aad.org/pamphlets/lichen.html

KERATOSES AND LEUKOPLAKIAS
Frictional keratosis
Frictional keratosis is quite common. It is caused by friction from the teeth or an appliance and is seen mainly on the alveolar ridge (Fig. 15) and may be seen at the occlusal line in the buccal mucosae, particularly in adult females – especially in those with temporomandibular pain-dysfunction syndrome.

Malignant change is rare but any sharp edges of teeth or appliances should be removed and the patient counselled about the habits.

Tobacco-induced keratoses
Tobacco is a common cause of keratosis, seen especially in males. The teeth are usually tar-stained and there may be mucosal smoker's

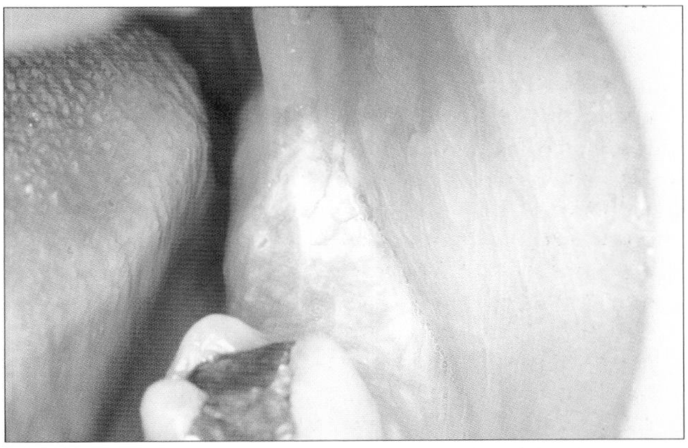

Fig. 15 Frictional keratosis, retromolar pad

Fig. 16 Frictional keratosis, lateral tongue

melanosis but malignant change is uncommon in most forms (Table 3).

Idiopathic keratoses
Many leukoplakias are uncommon and arise in the absence of any identifiable predisposing factors and most – up to 70% in large series – are benign without any evidence of dysplasia. However, the remaining 10–30% may be, or may become, either dysplastic or invasive carcinomas. Overall the rate of malignant transformation of all keratoses and leukoplakias is of some 3–6% over 10 years.

The lesions of greatest malignant potential are those leukoplakias which are:
- speckled, nodular or verrucous lesions (Figs 17 and 18)
- in at-risk sites (lateral tongue, ventral tongue, floor of mouth and soft palate complex) (Figs 19 and 20)
- associated with Candida (Fig. 6) or syphilis.

In these, rates of malignant transformation up to 30% have been reported in some series.

Diagnosis
The nature of white lesions can often only be established after further investigation.

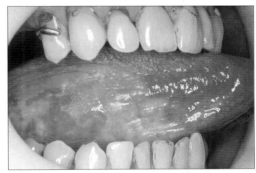

Fig. 17 Erythroleukoplakia

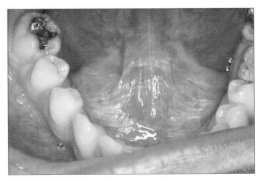

Fig. 18 Leukoplakia, floor of mouth

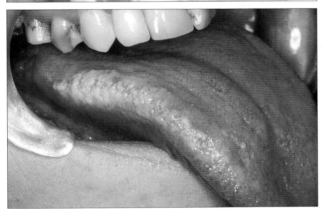

Table 3 Tobacco-induced keratoses

Tobacco habit	Common sites affected	Occasional sites affected	Malignant potential
Cigarette	lip (occasionally nicotine-stained) and commissures	Palate Others	Rare
Pipe smoking	palate (termed smoker's keratosis or stomatitis nicotina)	Others	Rare
Cigar	palate (termed smoker's keratosis or stomatitis nicotina)	Others	Rare
Snuff	gingival (together with recession)	Lip	Rare
Reverse smoking (Bidi) cigarettes are smoked with the lit end within the mouth	palate	Others	Common
Tobacco chewing	buccal	Others	Common

Biopsy is usually indicated, particularly where there is a high risk of malignant transformation, such as in lesions with:
- Any suggestion of malignancy
- Admixture with red lesions (speckled leukoplakia or erythroleukoplakia)
- A raised lesion (nodular or verrucous leukoplakia)

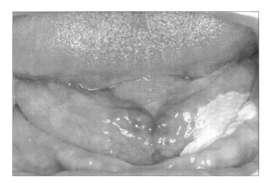

Fig. 19 Sublingual keratosis

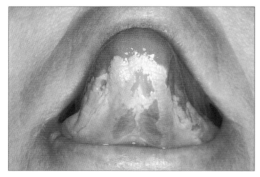

Fig. 20 Leukoplakia, ventral tongue, floor of mouth

- Candidal leukoplakia
- floor of mouth leukoplakia (sublingual keratosis)
- a rapid increase in size
- change in colour
- ulceration
- pain
- regional lymph node enlargement.

Prognosis

The finding by the pathologist of epithelial dysplasia may be predictive of malignant

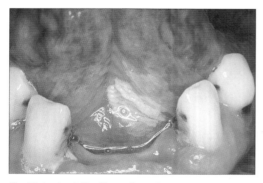

Fig. 21 Leukoplakia, floor of mouth

potential but this is not invariable, and there can be considerable inter- and intra-examiner variation in the diagnosis of dysplasia.

Thus there has been a search for molecular markers to predict exactly which lesions are truly of malignant potential and may develop into oral squamous cell carcinoma (OSCC).

The most predictive of the molecular or cellular markers thus far assessed for OSCC development apart from dysplasia, include chromosomal polysomy, the tumour suppressor p53 protein expression, and loss of heterozygosity (LOH) at chromosome 3p or 9p. Routine use of these is, however, hampered by their complexity and lack of facilities in many pathology laboratories.

Management

The dilemma in managing patients with potentially malignant oral lesions and field change has been of deciding which mucosal lesions or areas will progress to carcinoma. Specialist referral is indicated.

Cessation of dangerous habits such as tobacco and/or betel use (Figs 22 and 23), and the removal of lesions is probably the best course of action, particularly if they are the high-risk lesions or in a high risk group for carcinoma (see Chapter 9).

Perhaps surprisingly, management of leukoplakias is very controversial, since there are no randomised controlled double blind studies that prove the best type of treatment. Thus specialists may still offer

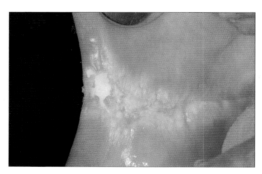

Fig. 22 Betel chewing keratosis

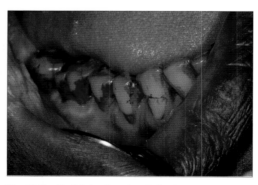

Fig. 23 Tooth staining from betel chewing

care which ranges from 'watchful waiting' to removal of the lesion (by laser, scalpel or other means) (Fig. 24).

Useful websites and patient information

http://www.cochrane.org/cochrane/revabstr/ab001829.htm
http://www.emedicine.com/ent/topic731.htm
http://www.mayoclinic.com/invoke.cfm?id=DS00458

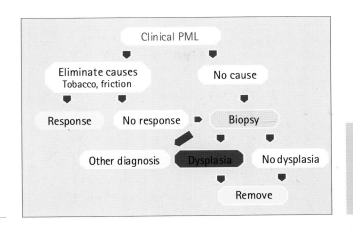

Fig. 24 Management of leukoplakias

Patients to refer

Keratoses which do not regress after elimination of aetiological factors

Hairy leukoplakia – if underlying cause of immunosuppression not already identified

Carcinoma

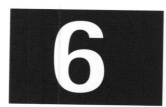
IN BRIEF

- Most red or hyperpigmented lesions in the mouth are inconsequential.
- However, cancer and some systemic diseases may present in this way.
- Most red lesions are inflammatory or atrophic but erthythroplasia is potentially malignant.
- Most hyperpigmented lesions are racial or due to embedded material (eg amalgam tattoo) but malignant and systemic disease can present in this way.
- Biopsy may be indicated.

Red and pigmented lesions

RED AND PIGMENTED LESIONS

This chapter covers red lesions and hyperpigmentation.

RED ORAL LESIONS

Red oral lesions are commonplace and usually associated with inflammation in, for example, mucosal infections. However, red lesions can also be sinister by signifying severe dysplasia in erythroplasia, or malignant neoplasms (Table 1).

Geographic tongue (*erythema migrans*)

Geographic tongue (Fig. 1) is a very common condition and cause of sore tongue, affecting at least 1-2% of patients. There is a genetic background, and often a family history. Many patients with a fissured tongue (scrotal tongue) also have geographic tongue. Erythema migrans is associated with psoriasis in 4% and the histological appearances of both conditions are similar. Some patients have atopic allergies such as hay fever and a few relate the symptoms to various foods. A few have diabetes mellitus.

Clinical features

Geographic tongue typically involves the dorsum of the tongue, sometimes the ventrum. It is often asymptomatic but a small minority of patients complain of soreness; these patients are virtually invariably middle-aged. If sore, this may be noted especially with acidic foods (for example tomatoes or citrus fruits) or cheese.

There are irregular, pink or red depapillated maplike areas, which change in shape, increase in

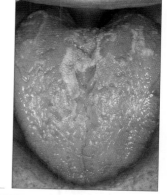

Fig. 1 Geographic tongue

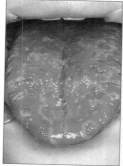

Figs 2 and 3 Geographic tongue

size, and spread or move to other areas sometimes within hours (Figs 2 and 3).

The red areas are often surrounded by distinct yellowish slightly raised margins. There is increased thickness of the intervening filiform papillae.

Table 1 Most common causes of red lesions

Localised

Inflammatory lesions

    Geographic tongue

    Candidosis

    Lichen planus

    Drugs

    Reactive lesions

    Pyogenic granulomas

    Peripheral giant cell granulomas

    Atrophic lesions

    Geographic tongue

    Lichen planus

    Lupus erythematosus

    Erythroplasia

    Avitaminosis B12

    Purpura

    Trauma

    Thrombocytopenia

    Vascular

    Telangiectases (Hereditary haemorrhagic telangiectasia or scleroderma or post-irradiation angiomas)

    Neoplasms

    Squamous carcinoma

    Kaposi's sarcoma

    Giant cell tumour

    Wegener's granulomatosis

Generalised

Inflammatory lesions

Most red lesions are inflammatory, usually geographic tongue (*erythema migrans*) (Figs 1 to 3)

Viral infections (eg herpes simplex stomatitis)

Fungal infections

Candidosis

    denture-related stomatitis, discussed below, is usually a form of mild chronic erythematous candidosis consisting of inflammation beneath a denture, orthodontic or other appliance (Fig. 4)

    median rhomboid glossitis; a persistent red, rhomboidal depapillated area in the midline dorsum of tongue (Fig. 5)

    acute oral candidosis; may cause widespread erythema and soreness sometimes with thrush, often a complication of corticosteroid or antibiotic therapy. Red lesions of candidosis may also be seen in HIV disease, typically in the palate (Fig. 6)

Bacterial infections:

Cancer treatment–related mucositis; common after irradiation of tumours of the head and neck, or chemotherapy eg for leukaemia

Immunological reactions such as lichen planus, plasma cell gingivostomatitis, granulomatous disorders (sarcoidosis, Crohn's disease, orofacial granulomatosis), amyloidosis, and graft versus host disease

Avitaminosis B or iron deficiency or folate deficiency

Diagnosis

The diagnosis of geographic tongue is clinical mainly from the history of a migrating pattern and the characteristic clinical appearance. Blood examination may rarely be nec-

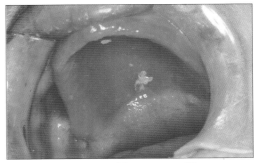

Fig. 4 Candida–associated denture stomatitis

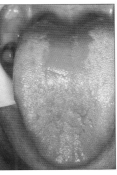

**Fig. 5
Median rhomboid glossitis**

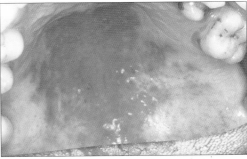

Fig. 6 Erythematous candidosis

essary to exclude diabetes, or anaemia if there is confusion with a depapillated tongue of glossitis.

Management

Reassurance remains the best that can be given. Zinc sulphate 200mg three times daily for three months or a topical rinse with 7% salicylic acid in 70% alcohol are advocated by some and may occasionally help.

Patient information and websites

http://www.usc.edu/hsc/dental/opath/Cards/GeographicTongue.html

http://www.worlddent.com/2001/05/series/ncuttic1_2.xml

DENTURE–RELATED STOMATITIS (DENTURE-INDUCED STOMATITIS; DENTURE SORE MOUTH; CHRONIC ERYTHEMATOUS CANDIDOSIS)

Denture-related stomatitis consists of mild inflammation of the mucosa beneath a denture — usually a complete upper denture. This is a common condition, mainly of the middle-aged or elderly, more prevalent in women than men.

Aetiopathogenesis

Dental appliances (mainly dentures) especially when worn throughout the night, or a dry mouth, favour development of this infection. It is not caused by allergy to the dental material (if it were, it would affect mucosae other than just that beneath the appliance).

However, it is still not clear why only some denture wearers develop denture-related stomatitis, since most patients appear otherwise healthy.

Dentures can produce a number of ecological changes; the oral flora may be altered and plaque collects between the mucosal surface of the denture and the palate.

The accumulation of microbial plaque (bacteria and/or yeasts) on and attached to the fitting surface of the denture and the underlying mucosa produces an inflammatory reaction. When candida is involved, the more common terms 'candida-associated denture stomatitis', 'denture-induced candidosis' or 'chronic erythematous candidosis' are used.

In addition, the saliva that is present between the maxillary denture and the mucosa may have a lower pH than usual. Denture-related stomatitis is sometimes associated also with various bacteria but is not exclusively associated with infection, and occasionally mechanical irritation is at play. Acrylic allergy is rarely a cause.

Clinical features

The characteristic presenting features of denture-related stomatitis are chronic erythema and oedema of the mucosa that contacts the fitting surface of the denture (Fig. 2). Uncommon complications include:
- Angular stomatitis
- Papillary hyperplasia in the vault of the palate.

Classification

Denture-related stomatitis has been classified into three clinical types (Newton's types), increasing in severity:
- A localised simple inflammation or a pinpoint hyperaemia (Type I)
- An erythematous or generalised simple type presenting as more diffuse erythema involving part of or the entire, denture-covered mucosa (Type II)
- A granular type (inflammatory papillary hyperplasia) commonly involving the central part of the hard palate and the alveolar ridge (Type III).

Diagnosis

Denture-related stomatitis is a clinical diagnosis although it may be confirmed by microbiological investigations. In addition haematological and biochemical investigations may be appropriate to identify any underlying predisposing factors such as nutritional deficiencies, anaemia and diabetes mellitus in patients unresponsive to conventional management.

Management

The denture plaque and fitting surface is infested with micro-organisms, most commonly *Candida albicans* and therefore, to prevent recurrence,

Table 2 Management of denture-related stomatitis
• Denture hygiene measures
• Antifungal therapy (eg topical or systemic)
• If unresponsive to above, investigate for underlying predisposing factors

dentures should be left out of the mouth at night, and stored in an appropriate antiseptic which has activity against yeasts (Table 2).

Cleansers containing alkaline hypochlorites, disinfectants, or yeast lytic enzymes are most effective against candida. Chlorhexidine gluconate can also eliminate *C.albicans* on the denture surface and a mouthwash can reduce the palatal inflammation.

The mucosal infection is eradicated by brushing the palate with chlorhexidine mouthwash or gel, and using miconazole gel, nystatin pastilles, amphotericin lozenges or fluconazole, administered concurrently with an oral antiseptic such as chlorhexidine which has antifungal activity.

Patient information and website

http://www.emedicine.com/derm/topic642.htm

Neoplastic lesions; red neoplasms include:
- Peripheral giant cell tumours
- Angiosarcomas such as Kaposi's sarcoma—a common neoplasm in HIV/AIDS, appears in the mouth as red or purplish areas or nodules especially seen in the palate
- Squamous cell carcinomas
- Wegener's granulomatosis.

Vascular anomalies (angiomas and telangiectasia) include:
- Dilated lingual veins (varices) may be conspicuous in normal elderly persons
- Haemangiomas are usually small isolated developmental anomalies, or hamartomas (Figs 7-9)
- Telangiectasias – dilated capillaries – may be seen after irradiation and in disorders such as hereditary haemorrhagic telangiectasia and systemic sclerosis (Fig. 10)
- Angiomas are benign and usually congenital (Figs 7-10). In general most do not require any active treatment unless symptoms develop, in which case they can be treated by injection of sclerosing agents, cryosurgery, laser excision or surgical excision.

Vesiculobullous disorders

Erythema multiforme, pemphigoid and pemphigus may present as red lesions (see Chapter 2), especially localised oral purpura, which presents with blood blisters (Fig. 11). Specialist referral is usually indicated.

Reactive lesions

Reactive lesions that can be red are usually persistent soft lumps (Figs 12 and 13) which include:
- Pyogenic granulomas
- Peripheral giant cell granulomas

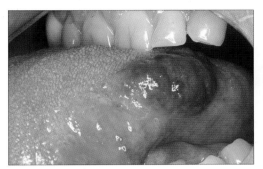

Fig. 7 Vascular hamartoma (haemangioma) tongue

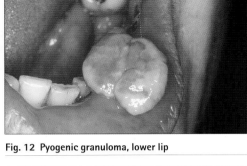

Fig. 12 Pyogenic granuloma, lower lip

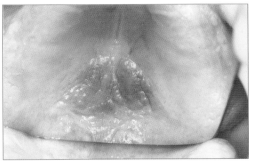

Fig. 8 Vascular hamartoma (haemangioma, palate)

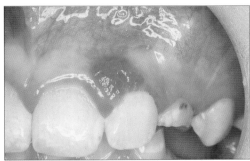

Fig. 13 Pyogenic epulis

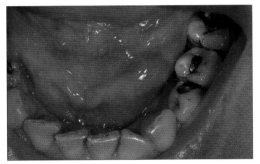

Fig. 9 Haemangioma in floor of mouth

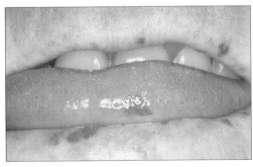

Fig. 10 Telangiectasia, lips and tongue

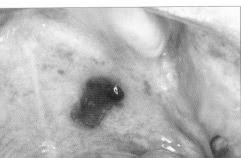

Fig. 11 Angina bullosa haemorrhagica

Specialist referral is usually indicated.

Atrophic lesions

The most important red lesion is erythroplasia, since it is often dysplastic (see below). Geographic tongue also causes red lesions (see above), desquamative gingivitis is a frequent cause of red gingivae, almost invariably caused by lichen planus or pemphigoid, and iron or vitamin deficiency states may cause glossitis (Fig. 14) or other red lesions.

ERYTHROPLAKIA (ERYTHROPLASIA)

Erythroplasia is a rare condition defined as 'any lesion of the oral mucosa that presents as bright red velvety plaques which cannot be characterised clinically or pathologically as any other recognisable condition'.

Mainly seen in elderly males, it is far less common than leukoplakia, but far more likely to be dysplastic or undergo malignant transformation.

Clinical features

Erythroplakia is seen most commonly on the soft palate, floor or mouth or buccal mucosa. Some erythroplakias are associated with white patches, and are then termed speckled leukoplakia or erythroleukoplakia (Fig. 15).

Diagnosis

Biopsy to assess the degree of epithelial dysplasia and exclude a diagnosis of carcinoma.

Prognosis

Erythroplasia has areas of dysplasia, carcinoma *in situ*, or invasive carcinoma in most cases. Carcinomas are seen 17 times more often in erythroplakia than in leukoplakia and these are therefore the most potentially malignant of all oral mucosal lesions.

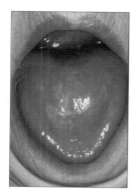

Fig. 14
Atrophic glossitis

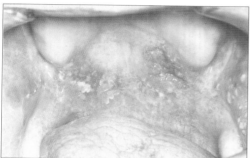

Fig. 15 Erythroleukoplasia in soft palate complex

Management

Erythroplastic lesions are usually (at least 85%) severely dysplastic or frankly malignant. Any causal factor such as tobacco use should be stopped, and lesions removed. There is no hard evidence as to the ideal frequency of follow-up, but it has been suggested that patients with mucosal potentially malignant lesions be re-examined within one month, at three months, at six months, at 12 months and annually thereafter.

PURPURA

This presents as bleeding into the skin and mucosa and is usually caused by trauma. Occasional small petechiae are seen at the occlusal line in perfectly healthy people.

Thrombocytopenia can result in red or brown pinpoint lesions (petechiae) or diffuse bruising (ecchymoses) at sites of trauma, such as the palate. Suction (eg fellatio) may produce bruising in the soft palate). Localised oral purpura or angina bullosa haemorrhagica is an idiopathic, fairly common cause of blood blisters, often in the soft palate, in older persons (Fig. 11). Sometimes the use of a corticosteroid inhaler precipitates this.

Diagnosis of red lesions

Diagnosis of red lesions is mainly clinical but lesions should also be sought elsewhere, especially on the skin or other mucosae.

It may be necessary to take a blood picture (including blood and platelet count), and assess haemostatic function or exclude haematinic deficiencies. Other investigations needed may include other haematological tests and/or biopsy or imaging.

Management

Treatment is usually of the underlying cause, or surgery.

HYPERPIGMENTATION

Oral mucosal discolouration may be superficial (extrinsic) or due to deep (intrinsic – in or beneath mucosa) causes and ranges from brown to black.

Extrinsic discolouration is rarely of consequence and is usually caused by:
- Habits such as tobacco or betel use
- Coloured foods or drinks, (such as liquorice, beetroot, red wine, coffee, tea)
- Drugs (such as chlorhexidine, iron salts, crack cocaine, minocycline, bismuth subsalicylate, and lansoprazole).

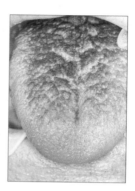

Fig. 16 Black hairy tongue

Black hairy tongue

This is one extrinsic type of discolouration seen especially in patients on a soft diet, smokers, and those with dry mouth or poor oral hygiene (Fig. 16).

The best that can usually be done is to avoid the cause where known, and to advise the patient to brush the tongue or use a tongue-scraper.

Intrinsic discolouration

This may have much more significance (Table 3). Localised areas of pigmentation may be caused mainly by:
- **Amalgam tattoo** (embedded amalgam). Typically this is a single blue-black macule in the mandibular gingiva close to the scar of an apicectomy (Figs 17 and 18) or where amalgam has accidentally been introduced into a wound, is painless, and does not change in size

Table 3 Main causes of intrinsic mucosal hyperpigmentation

Localised
- Amalgam or other tattoo
- Naevus
- Melanotic macule
- Neoplasms (eg malignant melanoma or Kaposi's sarcoma)
- Pigmentary incontinence
- Peutz-Jegher's syndrome

Generalised
- Racial pigmentation
- Localised irritation, eg tobacco or betel
- Drugs, eg antimalarials
- Pregnancy/oral contraceptive pill
- Addison's disease (hypoadrenocorticism)

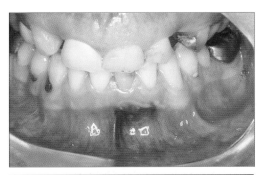

Fig. 17 Amalgam tattoo

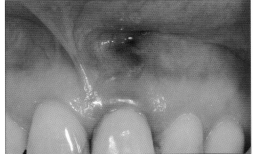

Fig. 18 Amalgam tattoo

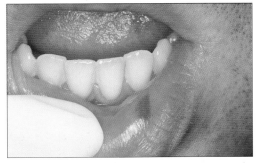

Fig. 19 Melanotic macule, lower labial mucosa

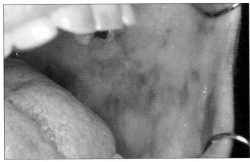

Fig. 20 Smoking-induced melanosis, buccal mucosa

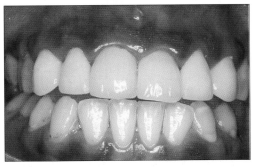

Fig. 21 Racial pigmentation

- **Naevi** are blue-black often papular lesions formed from increased melanin-containing cells (naevus cells) seen particularly on the palate. They are best removed to exclude melanoma.

- **Pigmentary incontinence** may be seen in some inflammatory lesions such as lichen planus, especially in smokers (Fig. 20).

- **Melanotic macules** are usually flat single brown, collections of melanin-containing cells, seen particularly on the vermilion border of the lip and on the palate (Fig. 19). They are best removed to exclude melanoma.

- **Malignant melanoma** is rare, seen usually in the palate or maxillary gingivae. Features suggestive of malignancy include a rapid increase in size, change in colour, ulceration, pain, the occurrence of satellite pigmented spots or regional lymph node enlargement. Incisional biopsy to confirm the diagnosis followed by radical excision is indicated.

- **Kaposi's sarcoma** is usually a purple lesion seen mainly in the palate or gingival of HIV-infected and other immunocompromised persons.

Generalised pigmentation, often mainly affecting the gingivae, is common in persons of colour, and is racial and due to melanin. Seen mainly in black and ethnic minority groups it can also be noted in some fairly light-skinned people (Fig. 21). Such pigmentation may be first noted by the patient in adult life and then incorrectly assumed to be acquired.

In all other patients with widespread intrinsic pigmentation, systemic causes should be excluded. These may include:
- Tobacco, which can also cause intrinsic hyper-pigmentation (smoker's melanosis)
- Antimalarials, oral contraceptive pill, anticonvulsants, minocycline, phenothiazines, gold, busulphan and other drugs
- Heavy metals (such as mercury, lead and bismuth) not used therapeutically now, rarely cause industrial exposure etc
- Pregnancy
- Hypoadrenalism (Addison's disease). Hyperpigmentation in this is generalised but most obvious in normally pigmented areas (eg the nipples, genitalia), skin flexures, and sites of trauma. The mouth may show patchy hyperpigmentation. Patients also typically have weakness, weight loss, and hypotension.

Diagnosis

The nature of oral hyperpigmentation can sometimes only be established after further investigation.

In patients with localised hyperpigmentation, in order to exclude melanoma,

or colour. A lesion suspected to be an amalgam tattoo is best radiographed first to see if there is radio-opaque material present, though not all are radio-opaque. If the lesion is not radio-opaque, it is best biopsied to exclude naevi or melanoma. Similar lesions can be caused by other foreign bodies (eg graphite tattoo), local irritation or inflammation.

radiographs may be helpful (they can sometimes show a foreign body) and biopsy may be indicated, particularly where there is a solitary raised lesion, a rapid increase in size, change in colour, ulceration, pain, evidence of satellite pigmented spots or regional lymph node enlargement. If early detection of oral melanomas is to be achieved, all pigmented oral cavity lesions should be viewed with suspicion. The consensus of opinion is that a lesion with clinical features as above seriously suggestive of malignant melanoma, are best biopsied at the time of definitive operation.

In patients with generalised or multiple hyperpigmentation, specialist referral is indicated.

Management
Management is of the underlying condition.

Patients to refer

Erythroplasia/erythroplakia — in view of high risk of malignant transformation

Squamous carcinoma

Isolated brown or black lesions of suspect aetiology

Generalised or multiple hyperpigmentation

Kaposi's sarcoma

Wegener's granulomatosis in view of associated systemic disease

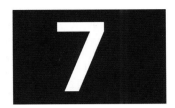

Disorders of orofacial sensation and movement

Sensory innervation of the mouth, face and scalp depends on the fifth cranial (trigeminal) nerve, so that lesions affecting this nerve can cause sensory loss or orofacial pain, or indeed both – sometimes with serious implications.

The facial (seventh cranial) nerve controls the muscles of facial expression, so that lesions of this nerve (lower motor neurone lesions) or its central connections (upper motor neurone lesions), can lead to facial weakness. The facial nerve also carries nerve impulses to the tear glands, to the salivary glands, and to the stapedius muscle of the stirrup bone (the stapes) in the middle ear and also transmits taste from the anterior tongue, so that lesions may also affect taste and hearing, lacrimation and salivation.

It is evident therefore that dental surgeons should be able to carry out examination of these and other cranial nerves (Table 1), as follows.

THE OLFACTORY NERVE (Ist CRANIAL NERVE)

Bilateral anosmia is common after head injuries, but in reality the patient may complain of loss of taste rather than sense of smell. Unilateral anosmia is often unnoticed by the patient.

An olfactory lesion is confirmed by inability to smell substances such as orange or peppermint oil. Ammoniacal solutions or other substances with a pungent odour must not be used since they stimulate the trigeminal rather than the olfactory nerve.

THE OPTIC NERVE (IInd CRANIAL NERVE)

Blindness or defects of visual fields are caused by ocular, optic nerve or cortical damage but the type of defect varies according to the site and extent of the lesion.

If there is a complete lesion of one optic nerve, that eye is totally blind and there is no direct reaction of the pupil to light (loss of constriction). If a light is shone into the affected eye, the pupil of the unaffected eye also fails to respond (loss of the consensual reflex). However, the nerves to the affected eye that are responsible for pupil constriction, run in the IIIrd cranial nerve and should be intact. If, therefore, a light is shone into the unaffected eye, the pupil of the affected eye also constricts even though it is sightless.

Lesions of the optic tract, chiasma, radiation or optic cortex cause various defects involving both visual fields but without total field loss on either side.

An ophthalmological opinion should always be obtained if there is any suggestion of a visual field defect.

THE OCULOMOTOR NERVE (IIIrd CRANIAL NERVE)

The oculomotor nerve supplies the muscle that raises the upper eyelid, most of the orbital muscles that move the eye (except the lateral rectus and superior oblique), and the ciliary muscle and pupil constrictor.

Normally the medial rectus (supplied by the IIIrd nerve) moves the eye medially (adducts). The lateral rectus (VIth nerve) abducts the eye. When the eye is abducted it is elevated by the superior rectus (IIIrd nerve) and depressed by the inferior rectus (IIIrd nerve). The adducted eye is depressed

Table 1 Examination of cranial nerves

	Nerve	Examination	Examination findings in lesions
I	Olfactory	Sense of smell	Impaired sense of smell for common odours (do not use ammonia)
II	Optic	Visual acuity Visual fields Pupil responses	Visual acuity reduced using Snellen types ± ophthalmoscopy: nystagmus. Visual fields by confrontation impaired; may be impaired pupil responses
III	Oculomotor	Eye movements Pupil responses	Diplopia; strabismus; eye looks down and laterally; movements impaired; ptosis; pupil dilated Pupil reactions: direct reflex impaired but consensual reflex intact
IV	Trochlear	Eye movements Pupil responses	Diplopia, particularly on looking down; strabismus; no ptosis; pupil normal and normal reactivity
V	Trigeminal	Sensation over face Corneal reflex Jaw jerk Taste sensation	Reduced sensation over face; ± corneal reflex impaired; ± taste sensation impaired; motor power of masticatory muscles reduced, with weakness on opening jaw; jaw jerk impaired; muscle wasting
VI	Abducens	Eye movements Pupil responses	Diplopia; strabismus; eye movements impaired to affected side; pupil normal and normal reactivity
VII	Facial	Motor power of facial muscles Corneal reflex Taste sensation	Impaired motor power of facial muscles on smiling, blowing out cheeks, showing teeth, etc; corneal reflex reduced; ± taste sensation impaired
VIII	Vestibulo-cochlear	Tuning fork at 256 Hz	Impaired hearing; impaired balance; ± nystagmus
IX	Glossopharyngeal	Gag reflex Taste sensation Voice	Reduced gag reflex; deviation of uvula; reduced taste sensation; voice may have nasal tone
X	Vagus	Gag reflex Voice	Reduced gag reflex; deviation of palate; voice hoarse
XI	Accessory	Ability to shrug shoulders and rotate head against resistance	Motor power of trapezius and sternomastoid reduced
XII	Hypoglossal	Tongue protrusion	Motor power of tongue impaired, with abnormal speech; ± fasciculation, wasting, ipsilateral deviation on protrusion

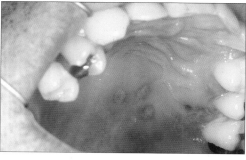

Fig. 1 Herpes zoster, palate

by the superior oblique muscle (IVth nerve) and elevated by the inferior oblique (IIIrd nerve).

Disruption of the oculomotor nerve therefore causes:
1. Ptosis (drooping upper eyelid).
2. Double vision (diplopia) and divergent squint (strabismus). The affected eye points downwards and laterally—'down and out' in all directions except when looking towards the affected side.
3. Paralysis of internal, upward and downward rotation of the eye.
4. A dilated pupil which fails to constrict on accommodation or when light is shone either onto the affected eye (negative direct light reaction) or into the unaffected eye (negative consensual light reaction).

THE TROCHLEAR NERVE (IVth CRANIAL NERVE)

The trochlear nerve supplies only the superior oblique muscle which moves the eye downwards and medially towards the nose.

The lesion is characterised by:
1. The head tilted away from the affected side.
2. Diplopia, maximal on looking downwards and inwards.
3. Normal pupils.

There is often damage to the IIIrd and VIth nerves as well.

Damage to the trochlear nerve causes serious disability, because there is diplopia maximal on looking down and the patient may therefore have difficulty reading, going down stairs or seeing obstructions on the ground.

THE TRIGEMINAL NERVE (Vth CRANIAL NERVE)

The trigeminal nerve supplies sensation over the whole face apart from the angle of the jaw, and the front of the scalp back to a line drawn across the vertex, between the ears. It also supplies sensation to the mucosae of the oral cavity, conjunctivae, nose, tympanic membrane and sinuses.

The motor division of the trigeminal nerve supplies the muscles of mastication (masseter, pterygoids, temporalis, mylohyoid and anterior belly of the digastric).

Taste fibres from the anterior two-thirds of the tongue, and secretomotor fibres to the submandibular and sublingual salivary glands and lacrimal glands, are also carried in branches of the trigeminal nerve.

Damage to a sensory branch of the trigeminal nerve causes hypoaesthesia in its area of distribution; infection such as with herpes zoster causes pain (Fig. 1). Lesions of the sensory part of the trigeminal nerve initially result in a diminishing response to pin-prick to the skin and, later, complete anaesthesia. Lesions involving the ophthalmic division also cause corneal anaesthesia: this is tested by gently touching the cornea with a wisp of cotton wool twisted to a point. Normally this procedure causes a blink (the corneal reflex), but not if the cornea is anaesthetised (and the patient does not see the cotton wool).

It is important, with patients complaining of facial anaesthesia, to test all areas but particularly the corneal reflex, and the reaction to pin-prick over the angle of the mandible.

If, however, the patient complains of complete facial or hemifacial anaesthesia, but the corneal reflex is retained or there is apparent anaesthesia over the angle of the mandible, then the symptoms are probably functional rather than organic.

Taste can be tested with sweet, salt, sour or bitter substances (sugar, salt, lemon juice or vinegar) carefully applied to the dorsum of the tongue.

Damage to the motor part of the trigeminal

nerve can be difficult to detect and is usually asymptomatic if unilateral but the jaw may deviate towards the affected side on opening. It is easier to detect motor weakness by asking the patient to open the jaw against resistance, rather than by trying to test the strength of closure.

THE ABDUCENS NERVE (VIth CRANIAL NERVE)

The abducens nerve supplies only one eye muscle, the lateral rectus. Lesions comprise:
1. Deviation of the affected eye towards the nose
2. Paralysis of abduction of the eye.
3. Convergent squint with diplopia maximal on looking laterally towards the affected side.
4. Normal pupils.

Lesions of the abducens can, however, be surprisingly disabling.

THE FACIAL NERVE (VIIth CRANIAL NERVE)

The facial nerve carries:
- The motor supply to the muscles of facial expression
- Taste sensation from the anterior two-thirds of the tongue (via the chorda tympani)
- Secretomotor fibres to the submandibular and sublingual salivary glands
- Secretomotor fibres to the lacrimal glands
- Branches to the stapedius muscle in the middle ear.

The neurones supplying the lower face receive upper motor neurones (UMN) from the contralateral motor cortex, whereas the neurones to the upper face receive bilateral UMN innervation.

An UMN lesion therefore causes unilateral facial palsy with some sparing of the frontalis and orbicularis oculi muscles because of the bilateral cortical representation. Furthermore, although voluntary facial movements are impaired, the face may still move with emotional responses, for example on laughing. Paresis of the ipsilateral arm (monoparesis) or arm and leg (hemiparesis), or dysphasia may be associated because of more extensive cerebrocortical damage.

Lower motor neurone (LMN) facial palsy is characterised by unilateral paralysis of all muscles of facial expression for both voluntary and emotional responses (Fig. 2). The forehead is unfurrowed and the patient unable to close the eye on that side. Attempted closure causes the eye to roll upwards (Bell's sign). Tears tend to overflow on to the cheek (epiphora), the corner of the mouth droops and the nasolabial fold is obliterated. Saliva may dribble from the commissure and may cause angular stomatitis. Food collects in the vestibule and plaque accumulates on the teeth on the affected side. Depending on the site of the lesion, other defects such as loss of taste or hyperacusis may be associated.

In facial palsy, facial weakness is demonstrated by asking the patient to:
- Close the eyes against resistance
- Raise the eyebrows

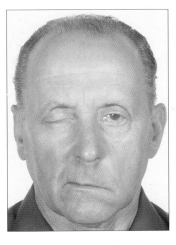

Fig. 2
Facial nerve palsy on the patient's left side

- Raise the lips to show the teeth
- Try to whistle.

Full neurological examination is needed, looking particularly for signs suggesting a central lesion, such as:
- Hemiparesis
- Tremor
- Loss of balance
- Involvement of the Vth, VIth or VIIIth cranial nerves.

The following investigations may be indicated:
- Imaging with MRI, or CT, of the internal auditory meatus, cerebellopontine angle and mastoid may be needed to exclude an organic lesion such as a tumour – particularly in progressive facial palsy
- Study of evoked potentials to assess the degree of nerve damage. Facial nerve stimulation or needle electromyography may be useful, as may electrogustometry, nerve excitability tests, electromyography and electroneuronography
- Blood pressure measurement (to exclude hypertension)
- Blood tests that may include:
  - Fasting blood sugar levels (to exclude diabetes)
  - Tests for HSV or other virus infections such as HIV may need to be considered
  - Full blood picture and haematinies as Crohn's disease may need to be considered
  - Serum angiotensin converting enzyme levels as a screen for sarcoidosis
  - Serum antinuclear antibodies to exclude connective tissue disease
  - In some areas, Lyme disease (tick-borne infection with *Borrelia burgdorferii*) should be excluded by ELISA test.
- Schirmer's test for lacrimation, carried out by gently placing a strip of filter paper on the lower conjunctival sac and comparing the wetting of the paper with that on the other side
- Test for loss of hearing
- Test for taste loss by applying sugar, salt, lemon juice or vinegar on the tongue and asking the patient to identify each of them
- Aural examination for discharge and other

signs of middle ear disease
- Blood pressure measurement (to exclude hypertension)
- Lumbar puncture occasionally.

THE VESTIBULOCOCHLEAR NERVE (VIIIth CRANIAL NERVE)

The auditory nerve has two components:
- The vestibular (concerned with appreciation of the movements and position of the head)
- The cochlear (hearing).

Lesions of this nerve may cause loss of hearing, vertigo or ringing in the ears (tinnitus).

An otological opinion should be obtained if a lesion of the vestibulocochlear nerve is suspected, as special tests are needed for diagnosis.

THE GLOSSOPHARYNGEAL NERVE (IXth CRANIAL NERVE)

The glossopharyngeal nerve carries:
- The sensory supply to the posterior third of the tongue and pharynx
- Taste sensation from the posterior third of the tongue
- Motor supply to the stylopharyngeus
- Secretomotor fibres to the parotid.

Symptoms resulting from a IXth nerve lesion include impaired pharyngeal sensation so that the gag reflex may be weakened; the two sides should always be compared. Lesions of the glossopharyngeal are usually associated with lesions of the vagus, accessory and hypoglossal nerves (bulbar palsy).

THE VAGUS NERVE (Xth CRANIAL NERVE)

The vagus has a wide parasympathetic distribution to the viscera of the thorax and upper abdomen but is also the motor supply to some soft palate, pharyngeal and laryngeal muscles.

Lesions of the vagus are rare in isolation but have the following effects:
1. Impaired gag reflex.
2. The soft palate moves towards the unaffected side when the patient is asked to say 'ah'.
3. Hoarse voice.
4. Bovine cough.

THE ACCESSORY NERVE (XIth CRANIAL NERVE)

The accessory nerve is the motor supply to the sternomastoid and trapezius muscles. Lesions are often associated with damage to the IXth and Xth nerves and cause:
1. Weakness of the sternomastoid (weakness on turning the head away from the affected side).
2. Weakness of the trapezius on shrugging the shoulders.

Testing this nerve is useful in differentiating patients with genuine palsies from those with functional complaints. In an accessory nerve lesion there is weakness on turning the head away from the affected side. Those shamming paralysis often simulate weakness when turning the head towards the 'affected' side.

THE HYPOGLOSSAL NERVE (XIIth CRANIAL NERVE)

The hypoglossal nerve is the motor supply to the muscles of the tongue. Lesions cause:
1. Dysarthria (difficulty in speaking) – particularly for lingual sounds.
2. Deviation of the tongue towards the affected side, on protrusion.

The hypoglossal nerve may be affected in its intra- or extracranial course. Intracranial lesions typically cause bulbar palsy. In an upper motor neurone lesion the tongue is spastic but not wasted; in a lower motor neurone lesion there is wasting and fibrillation of the affected side of the tongue.

FACIAL SENSORY LOSS

Normal facial sensation is important to protect the skin, oral mucosa and especially cornea from damage. Lesions developing and affecting the sensory part of the trigeminal nerve initially result in a diminishing response to light touch (cotton wool) and pin-prick (gently pricking the skin with a sterile pin or needle without drawing blood) and, later there is complete anaesthesia. Facial sensory awareness may be:
- Completely lost (anaesthesia) or
- Partially lost (hypoaesthesia).

The term paraesthesia does not mean loss of sensation, rather it means abnormal sensation.

Lesions of a sensory branch of the trigeminal nerve may cause anaesthesia in the distribution of the affected branch. Facial sensory loss may be caused by intracranial or, more frequently, by extracranial lesions of the trigeminal nerve and may lead to corneal, facial or oral ulceration (Table 2).

If the patient complains of complete facial or hemifacial anaesthesia, but the corneal reflex is retained then the symptoms are probably functional (non-organic) or due to benign trigeminal neuropathy. If the patient complains of complete facial or hemifacial anaesthesia and there is apparent anaesthesia over the angle of the mandible (an area not innervated by the trigeminal nerve) then the symptoms are almost certainly functional (non-organic).

Extracranial causes of sensory loss

Extracranial causes of facial sensory loss include damage to the trigeminal nerve from:
- Trauma, the usual cause
- Osteomyelitis and
- Malignant disease.

Common extracranial causes of facial sensory loss are shown in Table 2. The mandibular division or its branches may be traumatised by inferior alveolar local analgesic injections, fractures or surgery (particularly surgical extraction of lower third molars or osteotomies). Occasionally there is dehiscence of the mental foramen in an

Table 2 Causes of sensory loss in the trigeminal area

Extracranial

Trauma (eg surgical; fractures) to inferior dental, lingual, mental or infraorbital nerves

Inflammatory
- Osteomyelitis

Neoplastic
- carcinoma of antrum or nasopharynx
- metastatic tumours
- leukaemic deposits

Intracranial

Trauma (eg surgical; fractures or surgical treatment of trigeminal neuralgia)

Organic disease

Inflammatory
- multiple sclerosis
- neurosyphilis
- HIV infection
- sarcoidosis
- connective tissue diseases

Neoplastic
- cerebral tumours

Syringobulbia

Vascular
- cerebrovascular disease
- aneurysms

Drugs
- Labetalol

Bone disease
- Pagets disease
- Diabetes

Benign trigeminal neuropathy

Idiopathic

Psychogenic

Hysteria
- Hyperventilation syndrome

atrophic mandible leading to anaesthesia of the lower lip on the affected side, as a result of pressure from the denture. Osteomyelitis or tumour deposits in the mandible may affect the inferior alveolar nerve to cause labial anaesthesia.

Nasopharyngeal carcinomas may invade the pharyngeal wall to infiltrate the mandibular division of the trigeminal nerve, causing pain and sensory loss and, by occluding the Eustachian tube, deafness (Trotter's syndrome).

Damage to branches of the maxillary division of the trigeminal may be caused by trauma (middle-third facial fractures) or a tumour such as carcinoma of the maxillary antrum.

Intracranial causes of facial sensory loss

Intracranial causes of sensory loss are uncommon but serious and include:
- Multiple sclerosis
- Brain tumours
- Syringobulbia
- Sarcoidosis
- Infections (eg HIV).

Since other cranial nerves are anatomically close, there may be associated neurological deficits. In posterior fossa lesions for example, there may be cerebellar features such as ataxia. In middle cranial fossa lesions, there may be associated neurological deficits affecting cranial nerve VI (abducent nerve), resulting in impaired lateral movement of the eye.

Organic causes of facial sensory loss

These include diabetes or connective tissue disorders.

Benign trigeminal neuropathy

This is a transient sensory loss in one or more divisions of the trigeminal nerve which seldom occurs until the second decade. The corneal reflex is not affected. The aetiology is unknown, though some patients prove to have a connective tissue disorder.

Psychogenic causes of facial sensory loss

Hysteria, and particularly hyperventilation syndrome, may underlie some causes of facial anaesthesia.

Diagnosis in facial sensory loss

In view of the potential seriousness of facial sensory loss, care should be taken to exclude local causes and a full neurological assessment must be undertaken. Since, in the case of posterior or middle cranial fossa lesions, other cranial nerves are anatomically close, there may be associated neurological deficits . Thus in the absence of any obvious local cause, or if there are additional neurological deficits, patients should be referred for a specialist opinion.

Management of patients with facial sensory loss

If the cornea is anaesthetic, a protective eye pad should be worn and a tarsorrhaphy (an operation to unite the upper and lower eyelids) may be indicated since the protective corneal reflex is lost and the cornea may be traumatised.

OROFACIAL MOVEMENT DISORDERS

The facial nerve not only carries nerve impulses to the muscles of the face, but also to the salivary glands, to the lacrimal glands and to the stapedius muscle of the stirrup bone (the stapes) in the middle ear. It also transmits taste from the anterior tongue. Since the function of the facial nerve is so complex, several symptoms or signs may occur if it is disrupted.

The main movement disorder is facial palsy, which can have a range of causes (Table 3), and may be due to UMN or LMN lesions, as discussed above.

The common cause of facial palsy is stroke, an UMN lesions, and this is a medical emergency for which specialist care is indicated. The GDP should be able to differentiate UMN from LMN lesions (see above and Table 4).

The facial nerve should be tested, by examining facial movements and other functions mediated by the nerve. Movement of the mouth as the patient speaks is important, especially when they allow themselves the luxury of some emotional

ORAL MEDICINE

Key points for patients: Bell's palsy

- This is fairly common
- It affects only the facial nerve; there are no brain or other neurological problems
- It may be caused by herpes simplex virus, or other infections
- It is not contagious
- There are usually no serious long-term consequences
- X-rays and blood tests may be required
- Treatment takes time and patience; corticosteroids and antivirals can help
- Most patients recover completely within three months
- It rarely recurs

Key points for dentists: Bell's palsy

- This is fairly common
- It affects only the facial nerve
- It may be caused by herpes simplex virus, or other infections
- It is not contagious
- It disproportionately attacks pregnant women and people who have diabetes, hypertension, influenza, a cold, or immune problems
- There are usually no serious long-term consequences
- Corticosteroids and antivirals can help
- Most patients begin to get significantly better within two weeks, and about 80% recover completely within three months
- It rarely recurs, but can in 5-10%

Table 3 Causes of facial palsy

Upper motor neurone lesion
- Cerebrovascular accident
- Trauma
- Tumour
- Infection
- Multiple sclerosis

Lower motor neurone lesion
- Systemic infection
  - Bell's palsy (herpes simplex virus usually)
  - Varicella-Zoster virus infection (+/- Ramsay-Hunt syndrome)
  - Lyme disease (*B.burgdorferii*)
  - HIV infection
- Middle ear disease
  - Otitis media
  - Cholesteatoma
- Lesion of skull base
  - Fracture
  - Infection
- Parotid lesion
  - Tumour
  - Trauma to branch of facial nerve

Table 4 Differentiation of upper (UMN) from lower motor neurone (LMN) lesions of the facial nerve

	UMN lesions	LMN lesions
Emotional movements of face	Retained	Lost
Blink reflex	Retained	Lost
Ability to wrinkle forehead	Retained	Lost
Drooling from commissure	Uncommon	Common
Lacrimation, taste or hearing	Unaffected	May be affected

expression. The upper part of the face is bilaterally innervated and thus loss of wrinkles on one-half of the forehead or absence of blinking suggest a lesion is in the lower motor neurone.

If the patient is asked to close their eyes any palsy may become obvious, with the affected eyelids failing to close and the globe turning up so that only the white of the eye is showing (Bell's sign). Weakness of orbicularis muscles with sufficient strength to close the eyes can be compared with the normal side by asking the patient to close his eyes tight and observing the degree of force required to part the eyelids. If the patient is asked to wrinkle their forehead, weakness can be detected by the difference between the two sides.

Lower face (round the mouth) movements are best examined by asking the patient to:
- Smile
- Bare the teeth
- Purse the lips
- Blow out the cheeks
- Whistle.

Corneal reflex
This depends on the integrity of the trigeminal and facial nerve, either of which being defective will give a negative response. It is important to test facial light touch sensation in all areas but particularly the corneal reflex. Lesions involving the ophthalmic division cause corneal anaesthesia, which is tested by gently touching the cornea with a wisp of cotton wool twisted to a point. Normally, this procedure causes a blink but, if the cornea is anaesthetic (or if there is facial palsy), no blink follows, provided that the patient does not actually see the cotton wool.

Taste
Unilateral loss of taste associated with facial palsy indicates that the facial nerve is damaged proximal to the chorda tympani.

Hearing
Hyperacusis may be caused by paralysis of the stapedius muscle and this suggests the lesion is proximal to the nerve to stapedius.

Lacrimation
This is tested by hooking a strip of Schirmer or litmus paper in the lower conjunctival fornix. The strip should dampen to at least 15 mm in one minute if tear production is normal. The contralateral eye serves as a control (Schirmer's test). Secretion is diminished in proximal lesions of the facial nerve, such as those involving the geniculate ganglion or in the internal auditory meatus. It is reduced in Sjorgren's Syndrome (Chapter 3).

BELL'S PALSY
Bell's palsy is the most common acute LMN paralysis (palsy) of the face. There is inflammation of the facial nerve which may be immunologically mediated and associated with infection, commonly herpes simplex virus (HSV), leading to demyelination and oedema, usually in the stylomastoid canal.

The condition is usually seen in young adults; predisposing factors, found in a minority of cases, include:
- Pregnancy
- Hypertension
- Diabetes or
- Lymphoma.

Aetiopathogenesis
LMN facial palsy is usually associated with infections mainly with herpes simplex virus (HSV), rarely, another virus such as:
- Varicella-Zoster virus (VZV) infection
- Epstein-Barr virus (EBV) infection
- Cytomegalovirus (CMV) infection
- Human herpesvirus-6 infection
- HIV infection
- HTLV-1 infection;

occasionally with bacterial infections such as:
- Otitis media (middle ear infection)
- Lyme disease (infection with *Borrelia burgdorferii*) from camping or walking in areas that contain deer ticks.

Clinical features
Damage to the facial nerve may result in twitch-

ing, weakness, or paralysis of the face, in dryness of the eye or the mouth, or in disturbance of taste.

There is:
- Acute onset of paralysis over a few hours, maximal within 48 hours.
- Paralysis of upper and lower face, usually only unilaterally (Fig. 2).
- Diminished blinking and the absence of tearing. These together result in corneal drying, which can lead to erosion, and ulceration and the possible loss of the eye.

Occasionally:
- Pain around the ear or jaw may precede the palsy by a day or two.
- There may be apparent facial numbness, but sensation is actually intact on testing.

If the lesion is located proximal to the stylomastoid canal, there may also be (Table 5):
- Hyperacusis (raised hearing sensitivity; loss of function of nerve to stapedius), or
- Loss of taste (loss of function of the chorda tympani) and/or
- Loss of lacrimation.

Up to 10% of patients have a positive family history and a similar percentage suffers recurrent episodes.

Diagnosis of Bell's palsy

The history should be directed to exclude facial palsy caused by other factors, such as:
- Stroke
- Trauma to the facial nerve (eg in parotid region or to base of skull) or by underwater diving (barotrauma)
- Facial nerve tumours (eg acoustic neuroma)
- Facial nerve inflammatory disorders
- Multiple sclerosis
- Connective tissue disease
- Sarcoidosis
- Melkersson-Rosenthal syndrome
- Infections
(see page 40)

The examination and investigations are discussed above.

Management of Bell's palsy

Treatment with systemic corticosteroids results in 80-90% complete recovery. There is thus a strong argument for treating all patients with prednisolone 20mg four times a day for five days, then tailing off over the suc-

ceeding four days.

Since HSV is frequently implicated, antivirals are also justifiably used. The combination of oral aciclovir 400mg five times daily with oral prednisolone 1mg/kg daily for 10 days is more effective than corticosteroids alone.

WEBSITES AND PATIENT INFORMATION

http://www.entnet.org/bells.html
http://www.ninds.nih.gov/health_and_medical/disorders/bells_doc.htm
http://www.bellspalsy.ws/

Table 5 Localisation of site of lesion in and causes of unilateral facial palsy

Muscles paralysed	Lacrimation	Hyperacusis	Sense of taste	Other features	Probable site of lesion	Type of lesion
Lower face	N	No	N	Emotional movement retained + monoparesis or hemiparesis + aphasia	Upper motor neurone (UMN)	Stroke (cerebrovascular accident) Brain tumour Trauma HIV infection
All facial muscles	-	+	-	+ VIth nerve damage	Lower motor neurone (LMN) Facial nucleus	Multiple sclerosis
All facial muscles	-	+	-	+ VIIIth nerve damage	Between nucleus and geniculate ganglion	Fractured base of skull Posterior cranial fossa tumours Sarcoidosis
All facial muscles	N	+	N or -	No	Between geniculate ganglion and stylomastoid canal	Otitis media Cholesteatoma Mastoiditis
All facial muscles	N	No	N	No	In stylomastoid canal or extracranially	Bell's palsy Trauma Local analgesia (eg misplaced inferior dental block) Parotid malignant neoplasm Guillain-Barre syndrome
Isolated facial muscles	N	No	N	No	Branch of facial nerve extracranially	Trauma Local analgesia

N = normal   + = present   - = reduced

Patients to refer

Any patient with a cranial nerve defect as further investigation is outwith the scope of primary dental care

IN BRIEF
- Lumps have a variety of causes, benign and malignant.
- Biopsy, imaging or other investigations are often indicated.

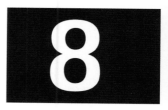

Lumps and swellings

This article discusses neck lumps, salivary gland swellings, and lumps and swellings in the mouth.

NECK LUMPS

The lymphoid system is the essential basis of immune defences and comprises predominantly bone marrow, spleen, thymus and lymph nodes too. Tissue fluid drains into lymph nodes which act as 'filters' of antigens and, after processing in the nodes, lymph containing various immunocytes drains from the nodes, to lymph ducts and then to the circulation. A lymph node consists of a cortex, paracortex and medulla and is enclosed by a capsule. Lymphocytes and antigens (if present) pass into the node through the afferent lymphatics, are 'filtered' and pass out from the medulla through the efferent lymphatics. The cortex contains B cells aggregated into primary follicles; following stimulation by antigen these develop a focus of active proliferation (germinal centre) and are termed secondary follicles. These follicles are in intimate contact with antigen-presenting dendritic cells. The paracortex contains T cells, and the medulla contains T and B cells.

Causes of cervical lymph node enlargement

Many diseases can present with lesions in the neck but the most common are lesions involving the lymph nodes (Table 1).

Nodes enlarge in oral infections or local infections in the drainage area (virtually anywhere in the head and neck). Most common is an enlarged jugulo-digastric (tonsillar) lymph node, inflamed secondary to a viral upper respiratory tract infection. Children and young adults are predominantly affected (Table 2). Enlarged cervical lymph nodes, especially in older people, may also be related to malignant disease in the drainage area (eg carcinoma) or may be a manifestation of systemic disease (eg HIV/AIDS) or leukaemia.

Examination of cervical lymph nodes

Inspection of the neck, looking particularly for swellings or sinuses, should be followed by careful palpation of the thyroid gland and all the lymph nodes, searching for swelling or tenderness.

The examination of lymph nodes in the neck is an important part of every orofacial examination. About one third of all the lymph nodes in the body are in the neck and dental surgeons can often detect serious disease through examining it.

It is prudent to adopt a systematic and methodical approach, examining different lymph node groups in turn:
- Submental
- Submandibular
- Pre-auricular/parotid
- Occipital
- Deep cervical chain.

Both anterior and posterior cervical nodes should be examined as well as other nodes, liver and spleen if systemic disease is a possibility. Most disease in lymph nodes is detected in the anterior triangle of neck, which is bounded superiorly by the mandibular lower border, posteriorly and inferiorly by the sternomastoid

Table 1 Causes of cervical lymph node enlargement

Inflammatory	Infective	Local	Bacterial	Local infections in the head and neck
			Viral	Viral respiratory infections Herpes simplex Herpes zoster Herpangina
		Systemic	Bacterial	Syphilis Tuberculosis Atypical mycobacterioses Cat scratch fever Brucellosis
			Viral	Glandular fever syndromes (EBV, CMV, HIV, HHV-6) Rubella
			Protozoal	Toxoplasmosis
			Others	Mucocutaneous lymph node syndrome (Kawasaki disease)
	Non-infective	Sarcoidosis Crohn's disease Orofacial granulomatosis Connective tissue diseases		
Malignancy	Primary	Leukaemias Lymphomas		
	Secondary	Metastases		
Other	Drugs, eg phenytoin			

Table 2 Lymph node swellings at different ages

Decade	Most common causes of swelling
First	Lymphadenitis due to viral respiratory tract infection
Second	Lymphadenitis due to viral respiratory tract infection Bacterial infection Glandular fever syndromes HIV infection Toxoplasmosis
Third and fourth	Lymphadenitis Glandular fever syndromes HIV infection Malignancy
After fourth	Lymphadenitis Malignancy

Table 3 Glandular fever syndromes

Features	Adolescents and young adults mainly	Sore throat, fever, lymphadenopathy		
Causal agents	Epstein-Barr virus (EBV)	Cytomegalovirus (CMV)	*Toxoplasma gondii*	Human immune deficiency viruses (HIV)
Investigations	Paul-Bunnell Test EBV antibody titres	CMV antibodies	Sabin-Feldman dye test Specific IgM antibodies	HIV antibody titres Lymphopenia T4 (CD4) cell numbers

drainage and nodes are then often firm, discrete and tender, but are mobile (lymphadenitis). The focus of inflammation can usually be found in the drainage area which is anywhere on the face, scalp and nasal cavity, sinuses, ears, pharynx and oral cavity. The local cause may not always be found despite a careful search. For example, children occasionally develop a *Staphylococcus aureus* lymphadenitis (usually in a submandibular node) in the absence of any obvious portal of infection. Lymph nodes that are tender may be inflammatory, leukaemia or lymphoma; those that are increasing in size and are hard may be malignant.

Lymph nodes may show reactive hyperplasia to a malignant tumour in the drainage area, or swelling because of metastatic infiltration. The latter may cause the node to feel distinctly hard, and it may become bound down to adjacent tissues ('fixed'), may not be discrete, and may even, in advanced cases, ulcerate through the skin. The neoplasms that frequently metastasise to cervical lymph nodes are oral squamous carcinoma (Chapter 9), nasopharyngeal carcinoma, tonsillar cancer and thyroid tumours.

Usually one or more anterior cervical nodes are involved, often unilaterally in oral neoplasms anteriorly in the mouth, but otherwise not infrequently bilaterally.

More serious is the finding of an enlarged node suspected to be malignant but where the primary neoplasm cannot be found. Nasopharyngeal or tonsillar carcinomas are classic causes of this and an ENT opinion should therefore be sought. Clinically unsuspected tonsillar cancer is a common cause of metastasis in a cervical node of unidentified origin. Biopsy of the tonsil may reveal a hitherto unsuspected malignancy.

Rare causes of cervical metastases include metastases from the stomach or even testicular tumours to lower cervical nodes. However, in some patients with a malignant cervical lymph node, the primary tumour is never located.

Generalised lymphadenopathy with or without enlargement of other lymphoid tissue such as liver and spleen (hepatosplenomegaly), suggests a systemic cause. Lymph nodes may swell when there are disorders involving the immune system more generally, such as the glandular fever syndromes, HIV/AIDS and related syndromes, various other viral infections; bacterial infections such as syphilis and tuberculosis; and parasites such as toxoplasmosis. In the systemic infective disorders the nodes are usually firm, discrete, tender and mobile. Lymph nodes may also swell in non infective lesions such as sarcoidosis; mucocutaneous lymph node syndrome (Kawasaki disease); and neoplasms such as lymphomas and leukaemias (Table 1). In the latter instances, and in the glandular fever syndromes including HIV (where there is lymphadenopathy often together with sore throat and fever; Table 3), there is usually enlargement of many or all cervical lymph nodes and in some there is involvement of the whole reticulendothelial system, with generalised lymph node enlargement

muscle, and anteriorly by the midline of the neck. Nodes in this site drain most of the head and neck except the occiput and back of neck. Lymphadenopathy in the anterior triangle of the neck alone is often due to local disease, especially if the nodes are enlarged on only one side.

A limited number of lymph nodes swell usually because they are involved in an immune response to an infectious agent in the area of (detectable clinically in neck, groin and axilla) and enlargement of the liver and spleen (hepatosplenomegaly). In the lymphomas particularly the nodes may be rubbery, matted together and fixed to deeper structures.

Management

A medical opinion is often indicated.

Salivary gland swelling

Salivary glands usually swell because of inflammation (sialadenitis), which is often viral but may have other causes (Table 4). Obstruction of salivary flow is another common cause (obstructive sialadenitis). Rare causes include salivary gland or other neoplasms.

In children, most salivary gland swellings are caused by mumps. In adults, most swellings of the salivary glands are caused by salivary duct obstruction (typically by a stone) but sialadenitis, Sjogren's syndrome and neoplasms are important causes to be excluded.

Diagnosis of salivary gland swelling

It can be difficult to establish whether a salivary gland is genuinely swollen, especially in obese patients. A useful guide to whether the patient is simply obese or has parotid enlargement is to observe the outward deflection of the ear lobe which is seen in true parotid swelling.

Diagnosis of the cause is mainly clinical but investigations such as imaging, liver function tests, serology for viral antibodies autoantibodies or biopsy, may be indicated.

Management

A specialist opinion is usually needed and treatment is of the underlying cause.

Immediate treatment is needed for acute bacterial sialadenitis; under ideal conditions antimicrobial therapy should be determined by results of culture and sensitivity of a sample of pus from the duct. However, as first line therapy, a penicil-

Table 4 Causes of salivary gland swelling

Inflammatory
   Mumps
   Ascending sialadenitis
   Recurrent parotitis
   HIV parotitis
   Other infections (eg tuberculosis)
   Sjogren's syndrome
   Sarcoidosis

Cystic fibrosis

Neoplasms (mainly pleomorphic salivary adenoma, but also monomorphic adenomas)

Duct obstruction (eg calculus)

Sialosis (usually caused by autonomic dysfunction in starvation, bulimia, diabetes, or alcoholic cirrhosis)

Deposits rarely

(eg amyloidosis and haemochromatosis)

Drugs rarely (eg chlorhexidine, methyl dopa, phenylbutazone, iodine compounds, thiouracil, catecholamines, sulfonamides, phenothiazines and protease inhibitors)

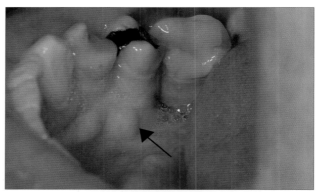

Fig. 1 Torus mandibularis

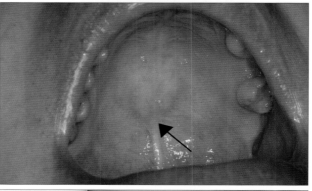

Fig. 2 Torus palatinus

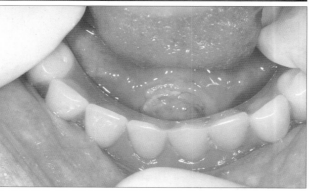

Fig. 3 Denture-induced hyperplasia and ulceration

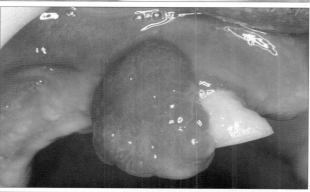

Fig. 4 Epulis

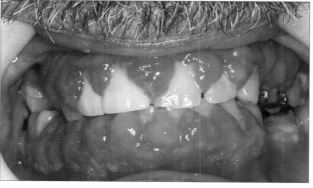

Fig. 5 Calcium channel blocker-induced gingival swelling

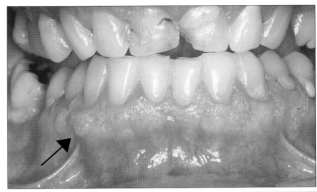

Fig. 6 Human papillomavirus infection

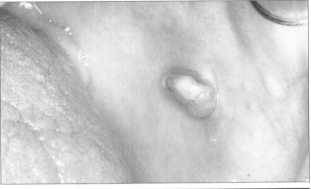

Fig. 7 Pyogenic granuloma

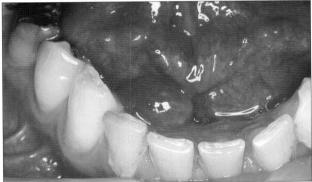

Fig. 8 Mucocoele in the floor of mouth (ranula)

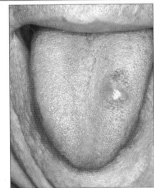

Fig. 9 Vascular hamartoma (haemangioma), dorsum of tongue

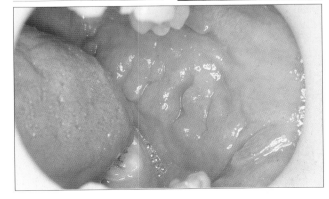

Fig. 10 Orofacial granulomatosis showing cobblestoning buccal mucosa

linase-resistant penicillin such as flucloxacillin is appropriate. In patients with penicillin allergy, erythromycin is a suitable alternative. In addition general supportive measures such as analgesia and increased fluid intake are important. Thereafter, specialist referral is generally indicated to identify any predisposing factors.

LUMPS AND SWELLINGS IN THE MOUTH

Lumps and swellings in the mouth are common, but of diverse aetiologies (Table 5) and some develop into ulcers, as in various bullous lesions (see Chapter 2) and in malignant neoplasms (see Chapter 9).

Many different conditions, from benign to malignant, may present as oral lumps or swellings (see tables) including:

- **Developmental**; unerupted teeth, and tori - congenital bony lumps lingual to the mandibular premolars (torus mandibularis; Fig. 1), or in the centre of the palate (torus palatinus; Fig. 2) are common causes of swellings related to the jaws.
- **Inflammatory**; dental abscess is one of the most common causes of oral swelling. However, conditions characterised by chronic inflammation and granulomas, which can present with lumps or swellings – these include Crohn's disease, orofacial granulomatosis (OFG), and sarcoidosis (discussed below).
- **Traumatic**; haematoma may cause a swelling at the site of trauma. The flange of a denture impinging on the vestibular mucosa may stimulate a reactive irregular hyperplasia (denture-induced hyperplasia) (Fig. 3).
- **Neoplasms**; benign epulides (Fig. 4) or malignant tumours such as oral squamous cell carcinoma (OSCC), Kaposi's sarcoma, lymphoma and other neoplasms may present as swellings, as discussed in Chapter 9. Occasionally, metastatic malignant disease may present as a lump.
- **Fibro-osseous lesions**; fibrous dysplasia and Paget's disease can result in hard jaw swellings.
- **Hormonal and metabolic**; pregnancy may result in a gingival swelling (pregnancy epulis)
- **Drug-induced**; a range of drugs can produce gingival swelling - most commonly implicated are phenytoin, calcium channel blockers and ciclosporin (Fig. 5).
- **Allergic lesions**; angioedema in particular can cause swellings.
- **Viral lesions**; papillomas, common warts (verruca vulgaris), and genital warts (condyloma acuminatum) are all among the lumps caused by human papillomaviruses (HPV; Fig. 6).

Causes of lumps and swellings according to site

Carcinomas and other malignant neoplasms (See Chapter 9) can present in any site.

Gingiva

Sometimes, hyperplasia is congenital. Rapidly developing localised lumps, usually associated

Table 5 Main conditions which may present as lumps or swellings in the mouth

Normal anatomy	Pterygoid hamulus Parotid papillae Lingual papillae (foliate and circumvallate)
Developmental	Unerupted teeth Odontogenic cysts Eruption cysts Developmental cysts (eg thyroglossal, dermoid) Haemangioma Lymphangioma Maxillary and mandibular tori Hereditary gingival fibromatosis Lingual thyroid
Inflammatory	Abscess Cellulitis Cysts Insect bites Sialadenitis Pyogenic granuloma Chronic granulomatous disorders Orofacial granulomatosis Crohn's disease Sarcoidosis
Traumatic	Denture granuloma Epulis Fibroepithelial polyp Haematoma Mucocele Surgical emphysema
Neoplasms	Carcinoma Leukaemia Lymphoma Myeloma Odontogenic tumours Minor salivary glands Others
Fibro-osseous	Cherubism Fibrous dysplasia Paget's disease
Hormonal	Pregnancy epulis/gingivitis Oral contraceptive pill gingivitis
Metabolic	Amyloidosis Other deposits
Drugs	Phenytoin Calcium channel blockers Ciclosporin
Allergic	Angioedema
Infective	HPV

Table 6 Main features of OFG

- Ulcers
- Facial or labial swelling
- Angular cheilitis
- Lip fissures
- Mucosal tags
- 'Cobblestone' proliferation of the mucosa
- Gingival swelling

with discomfort, are most likely to be abscesses, usually a dental abscess. Other localised swellings are usually inflammatory, such as the pyogenic granuloma (Fig. 7) or neoplastic.

Most generalised gingival swellings are due to hyperplasia with oedema related to plaque deposits, occasionally exacerbated by hormonal changes (puberty, pregnancy) or drugs. Such changes often develop slowly – over weeks rather than days – and are usually without discomfort.

There are very few serious causes of generalised enlargements of the gingivae appearing spontaneously or rapidly, but leukaemia is one prime example.

Palate

Lumps of the hard palate may develop from structures within the palate (intrinsic) or beyond it (extrinsic). Thus, for example, torus palatinus (Fig. 2) is an intrinsic bone lesion, whereas a dental abscess pointing on the palate (usually from the palatal roots of the first and second maxillary molars, or from upper lateral incisors) is extrinsic. Unerupted teeth, especially permanent canines, or second premolars are relatively common. Other causes of palatal swellings are uncommon but it should be remembered that the palate is the second most common site (after the parotid) for pleomorphic adenomas and other salivary neoplasms. Invasive carcinoma from the maxillary sinus may produce a palatal swelling. Kaposi's sarcoma, typical of HIV/AIDS, may also present as a lump in the palate, or elsewhere. Developing unilateral hard palatal swellings, characteristically disturbing the fit of an upper denture in older patients, may denote Paget's disease.

Floor of mouth

Swellings in the floor of the mouth are more likely to arise from structures above the mylohyoid muscle than below it. The commonest swellings in the floor of the mouth are denture-induced hyperplasia (Fig. 3) or a salivary calculus.

Other lesions producing swellings in this area are a mucocele (known as ranula because of the resemblance to a frog's belly; Fig. 8) and neoplasms of the sublingual salivary gland (usually malignant), but these are relatively uncommon. Patients occasionally describe a lump which proves to be a swelling of the lingual aspect of the mandible (more characteristic of ameloblastoma than of dental abscesses or cysts). Swellings of the submandibular salivary gland and adjacent lymph nodes may occasionally be described by patients as being in the floor of the mouth. However, only very large swellings below the mylohyoid muscle are likely to produce a bulge in the mouth. Swellings in the floor of the mouth may inhibit swallowing and talking.

Mandibular tori (Fig. 1) produce bony hard swellings lingual to the lower premolars.

Tongue and buccal mucosa

Discrete lumps may be of various causes – congenital (Fig. 9; haemangioma), inflammatory, traumatic or neoplastic.

The tongue may be congenitally enlarged (macroglossia) in, for example, Down syndrome, or may enlarge in angioedema, gigantism, acromegaly or amyloidosis.

Causes of swellings include haematomas from trauma (such as occasional biting), infections, angioedema, fibro-epithelial polyps, fibrous lumps, mucoceles (Fig. 9), vesiculobullous lesions, and occasionally insect bites.

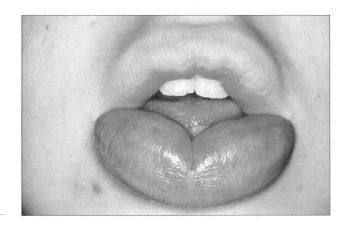

Fig. 11 Orofacial granulomatosis with chronic lip swelling

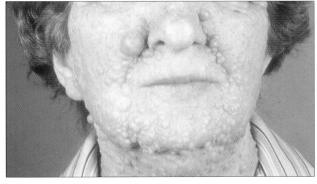

Fig. 12 Neurofibromatosis, face

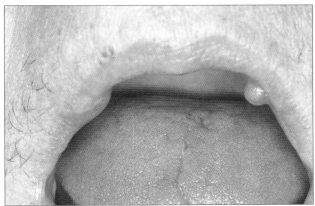

Fig. 13 Neurofibromatosis, upper lip

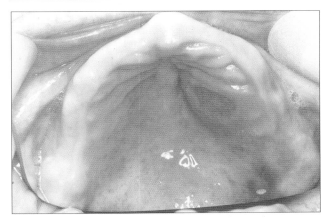

Fig.14 Minor salivary gland neoplasm

Systemic conditions such as Crohn's disease, orofacial granulomatosis and occasionally sarcoid may produce widespread irregular thickening (cobblestoning) of the cheek mucosa (Fig. 10) or the lips (Fig. 11).

Some 'lumps' become ulcers, as in various bullous lesions, in primary and tertiary syphilis and in malignant neoplasms.

The flange of a denture impinging on the vestibular mucosa may stimulate a reactive irregular hyperplasia – the so-called denture granuloma or denture-induced hyperplasia (Fig. 3). Salivary neoplasms in the lip may simulate, but are usually harder than, mucous cysts. Mucoceles are uncommon in the upper lip; discrete swellings there may well be salivary gland neoplasms.

Diagnosis of the cause of a lump or swelling

When patients refer to a lump in the mouth it is important to establish when it was first noticed. The tongue often detects even very small swellings and patients may also notice a lump because it is sore. Most patients have only a passing interest in their mouths but some examine their mouths out of idle curiosity, some through fear (perhaps after hearing of someone with 'mouth cancer'). Indeed it is not unknown for some individuals (including dental staff!) to discover and worry about the parotid papilla, foliate papillae on the tongue, or the pterygoid hamulus. The medical history should be fully reviewed, and there should be a thorough examination, since some systemic disorders may be associated with intra-oral or facial swellings (Figs. 12 and 13).

Features of a lump which can be diagnostically useful are:

a) The number of lesions – particularly with regard to whether the lesion is bilaterally symmetrical and thus possibly anatomical;

b) Alteration in size;

c) Any discharge from the lesion (clear fluid, pus, blood).

d) When patients refer to a lump in the mouth, it is important to establish when it was first noticed.

Important features to consider when making the provisional diagnosis of the cause of a lump or swelling include:

- Position. The anatomical position should be defined and the proximity to other structures (eg teeth) noted.
- Midline lesions tend to be developmental in origin (eg torus palatinus).
- Bilateral lesions tend to be benign (eg sialosis – salivary swelling in alcoholism, diabetes or other conditions).
- Most neoplastic lumps are unilateral (Fig. 14).

Other similar or relevant changes elsewhere in the oral cavity should be noted.

- Size. The size should always be measured and recorded. A diagram or photograph may be helpful.
- Shape. Some swellings have a characteristic shape which may suggest the diagnosis: thus a parotid swelling often fills the space between the posterior border of the mandible and the mastoid process.
- Colour. Brown or black pigmentation may be due to a variety of causes such as a tattoo, naevus or melanoma. Purple or red may be

due to a haemangioma (Fig. 9), Kaposi's sarcoma or giant-cell lesion.

- Temperature. The skin overlying acute inflammatory lesions, such as an abscess, or a haemangioma, is frequently warm.
- Tenderness. Inflammatory swellings such as an abscess are characteristically tender, although clearly palpation must be gentle to avoid excessive discomfort to the patient.
- Discharge. Note any discharge from the lesion (eg clear fluid, pus, or blood), orifice, or sinus.
- Movement. The swelling should be tested to determine if it is fixed to adjacent structures or the overlying skin/mucosa — such as may be seen with a neoplasm.
- Consistency. Palpation showing a hard (indurated) consistency may suggest a carcinoma. Palpation may cause the release of fluid (eg pus from an abscess) or cause the lesion to blanch (vascular) or occasionally cause a blister to appear (Nikolsky sign) or to expand. Sometimes palpation causes the patient pain (suggesting an inflammatory lesion). The swelling overlying a bony cyst may crackle (like an egg-shell) when palpated or fluctuation may be elicited by detecting movement of fluid when the swelling is compressed. Palpation may disclose an underlying structure (eg the crown of a tooth under an eruption cyst) or show that the actual swelling is in deeper structures (eg submandibular calculus).
- Surface texture. The surface characteristics should be noted: papillomas have an obvious anemone-like appearance (Fig. 6); carcinomas and other malignant lesions tend to have a nodular surface and may ulcerate. Abnormal blood vessels suggest a neoplasm.
- Ulceration. Some swellings may develop superficial ulceration such as squamous cell carcinoma. The character of the edge of the ulcer and the appearance of the ulcer base should also be recorded.
- Margin. Ill-defined margins are frequently associated with malignancy, whereas clearly defined margins are suggestive of a benign lesion.
- Number of swellings. Multiple lesions suggest an infective or occasionally developmental, origin. Some conditions are associated with multiple swellings of a similar nature, eg neurofibromatosis (Figs 12 and 13).

Investigations

The nature of many lumps cannot be established without further investigation.

- Any teeth adjacent to a lump involving the jaw should be tested for vitality, and any caries or suspect restorations investigated.
- The periodontal status of any involved teeth should also be determined.
- Imaging of the full extent of the lesion and possibly other areas is required whenever lumps involve the jaws. OPT and special radiographs (eg of the skull, sinuses, salivary gland function), computerised tomography (CT scans) or magnetic resonance imaging (MRI), or ultrasound may, on occasions, be indicated. Photographs may be useful for future comparison.
- Blood tests may be needed, particularly if there is suspicion that a blood dyscrasia or endocrinopathy may underlie the development of the lump.
- Biopsy is often required especially if the lesion is single and chronic, since it may be a neoplasm (Fig. 14) or other serious condition.

CHRONIC GRANULOMATOUS CONDITIONS

There are a number of patients who present with chronic swellings or lumps, which on biopsy prove to have histological evidence of non-caseating epithelioid cell granulomas. These conditions include orofacial granulomatosis, Crohn's disease, and sarcoidosis.

Orofacial granulomatosis

Orofacial granulomatosis (OFG) is an uncommon but increasingly recognised condition seen mainly in adolescents and young adults which usually manifests with chronic facial and/or labial swelling, but which can also manifest with angular stomatitis and/or cracked lips, ulcers, mucosal tags, mucosal cobble-stoning, or gingival swelling (Figs 10 and 11; Table 6).

Some patients with similar features have, or develop, gastrointestinal Crohn's disease or sarcoidosis.

The aetiology of OFG is unknown but in some there is a postulated reaction to food or other antigens (particularly to additives/preservatives such as benzoates or cinnamaldehyde), or metals such as cobalt. Most patients appear to develop the problem in relation to dietary components such as chocolate, nuts, cheese or food additives.

Conditions related to OFG include Miescher's cheilitis – where lip swelling is seen in isolation, and Melkersson-Rosenthal syndrome – where there is facial swelling with fissured tongue and recurrent facial palsy.

Diagnosis

Diagnosis is clinical, supported by blood tests, endoscopy, imaging and biopsy to differentiate from Crohn's disease, sarcoidosis, tuberculosis and foreign body reactions. Specialist care is usually indicated.

Management

Management is to eliminate allergens such as chocolate, nuts, cheese, cinnamaldehyde or food additives and treat lesions with intralesional corticosteroids or occasionally topical tacrolimus, systemic clofazimine or sulfasalazine.

Useful websites

http://www.emedicine.com/derm/topic72.htm

Crohn's disease

Crohn's disease is a chronic inflammatory idiopathic granulomatous disorder. Many causal factors have been hypothesised but not proved.

Crohn's disease affects mainly the small intestine (ileum) but can affect any part of the gastrointestinal tract, including the mouth.

About 10% of patients with Crohn's disease of the bowel have oral lesions. Oral lesions may be seen in the absence of any identifiable gut involvement and are the same as those seen in OFG — reddish raised lesions on the gingiva, hyperplastic folds of the oral mucosa (thickening and folding of the mucosa producing a 'cobblestone type' of appearance, and mucosal tags), ulcers (classically linear vestibular ulcers with flanking granulomatous masses), facial swelling and angular cheilitis. There may also be features of gastrointestinal involvement such as abnormal bowel movements, abdominal pain, rectal bleeding or weight loss.

Diagnosis
Oral biopsy, haematological, gastrointestinal and other investigations may be required in suspected Crohn's disease especially to exclude sarcoidosis. Specialist care is usually indicated. Histologically, the epithelium is intact but thickened, with epithelioid cells and giant cells surrounded by a lymphocytic infiltration.

Management
Topical or intralesional corticosteroids or topical tacrolimus may effectively control the oral lesions but more frequently systemic corticosteroids, azathioprine or salazopyrine are required.

Sarcoidosis
Sarcoidosis is a multi-system granulomatous disorder, of unclear aetiology, which most commonly affects young adult females, especially Afro-Caribbeans.

Sarcoidosis typically causes bilateral hilar lymphadenopathy, pulmonary infiltration and impaired respiratory efficiency, skin and eye lesions but can involve virtually any tissue. Because of its vague and protean manifestations, sarcoidosis appears to be under-diagnosed. Gingival enlargement, or oral swellings may be seen but sarcoidosis can involve any of the oral tissues and has a predilection for salivary glands, causing asymptomatic enlargement of the major salivary glands and some have xerostomia. The association of salivary and lacrimal gland enlargement with fever and uveitis is known as uveoparotid fever (Heerfordt's syndrome).

Diagnosis
The most helpful investigations include:
- Chest radiography (for enlarged hilar lymph nodes)
- Raised levels of serum angiotensin-converting enzyme (SACE) in acute disease
- A positive gallium or PET (positron emission tomography) scan of lacrimal and salivary glands
- Labial salivary gland biopsy (for histological evidence of non-caseating epithelioid cell granulomas).

Management
Patients with sarcoidosis but only minor symptoms often require no treatment. If there is active ocular disease, progressive lung disease, hypercalcaemia, or cerebral involvement or other serious complications, corticosteroids are given.

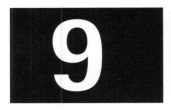

IN BRIEF
- Oral cancer is increasing in young people.
- Tobacco and alcohol are the most common aetiological factors.
- Any lump or ulcer lasting more than three weeks should be regarded with suspicion.
- Surgery and radiotherapy are the main treatments.

Oral cancer

ORAL CANCER

Oral cancer is the most common malignant epithelial neoplasm affecting the mouth. More than 90% is oral squamous cell carcinoma (OSCC) (Table 1).

Table 1 Oral malignant neoplasms
Common
Oral squamous cell carcinoma
Cancers of the oral cavity are classified according to site:
• lip (International Classification of Diseases (ICD) 140),
• tongue (ICD 141),
• gum (ICD 143),
• floor of the mouth (ICD 144) and
• unspecified parts of the mouth (ICD 145)
Less common
• Kaposi's sarcoma
• Lymphoma
• Malignant melanoma
• Maxillary antral carcinoma (or other neoplasms)
• Metastatic neoplasms (breast, lung, kidney, stomach, liver)
• Neoplasms of bone and connective tissue
• Odontogenic tumours
• Salivary gland tumours
• Others

Oral squamous cell carcinoma (OSCC) is among the 10 most common cancers worldwide. The number of new mouth (oral) and oropharyngeal cancers is currently estimated to be 300,000 cases worldwide, amounting to around 3% of total cancers. In the UK, the total number of recorded cases of oral cancer is about 4,500, with around 1,700 deaths, and the incidence appears to be rising in the UK and many other countries. In the UK, there was a 17% increase in cases of oral cancer from 3,673 in 1995 to 4,304 in 1999. Scotland has about double the incidence rate of oral cancer compared with England. The mortality rate in the UK is just over 50%, despite treatment.

OSCC is seen predominantly in males but the male:female differential is decreasing. OSCC is seen predominantly in the elderly but is increasing in younger adults.

POTENTIALLY MALIGNANT STATES

Some potentially malignant (precancerous) lesions which can progress to OSCC include the following (Table 2):
- Erythroplasia (erythroplakia; see Chapter 6) – this is the lesion most likely to progress to carcinoma, and is very dangerous.
- Leukoplakias (See Chapter 5), particularly:
  - Nodular leukoplakia
  - Speckled leukoplakia
  - Proliferative verrucous leukoplakia
  - Sublingual leukoplakia
  - Candidal leukoplakia
  - Syphilitic leukoplakia.

Some other potentially malignant (precancerous) conditions include:
- Actinic cheilitis (from ultraviolet light expo-

sure - mainly seen on the lower lip)
- Lichen planus (mainly the non-reticular or erosive type)
- Submucous fibrosis (seen in users of areca nut)
- Rarities such as:
  - Dyskeratosis congenita
  - Discoid lupus erythematosus
  - Paterson-Kelly syndrome (sideropenic dysphagia; Plummer-Vinson syndrome).

Table 2 Potentially malignant oral lesions

Lesion	Aetiology	Features
Erythroplasia	Tobacco/alcohol	Flat red plaque
Leukoplakia	Tobacco/alcohol	White or speckled plaque
Proliferative verrucous leukoplakia	Tobacco/alcohol/ human papillomavirus (HPV)	White or speckled or nodular plaque
Sublingual keratosis	Tobacco/alcohol	White plaque
Actinic cheilitis	Sunlight	White plaque/erosions
Lichen planus	Idiopathic	White plaque/erosions/red lesions
Submucous fibrosis	Areca nut	Immobile mucosa
Discoid lupus erythematosus	Idiopathic	White plaque/erosions/red lesions
Chronic candidosis	Candida albicans	White or speckled plaque
Syphilitic leukoplakia	Syphilis	White plaque
Atypia in immunocompromised patients	HPV	White or speckled plaque
Dyskeratosis congenita	Genetic	White plaques
Paterson-Kelly syndrome (sideropenic dysphagia; Plummer-Vinson syndrome)	Iron deficiency	Post-cricoid web

PREDISPOSING FACTORS (RISK FACTORS)

OSCC is most common in older males, in lower socioeconomic groups and in ethnic minority groups.

OSCC arises because of damage to DNA (mutations) which can arise spontaneously, probably because of free radical damage, or can be caused by chemical mutagens (carcinogens), ionising radiation or micro-organisms. OSCC arises as a consequence of multiple molecular events causing genetic damage affecting many chromosomes and genes, and leading to DNA changes. The accumulation of genetic changes leads to cell dysregulation to the extent that growth becomes autonomous and invasive mechanisms develop – this is carcinoma (Fig. 1).

Actinic radiation may predispose to lip cancer but the hazards from other types of radiation are unclear.

Intraoral squamous cell carcinoma (OCC) is seen especially in relation to various lifestyle habits. These are mainly tobacco and alcohol related.

Tobacco, whether smoked or chewed, releases a complex mixture of at least 50 compounds including polycyclic aromatic hydrocarbons such as benzpyrene, nitrosamines, aldehydes and aromatic amines which are carcinogens.

Alcohol (ethanol) is metabolised to acetaldehyde, which may be carcinogenic. Nitrosamine and urethane contaminants may also be found in some alcoholic drinks. Alcohol damage to the liver might, by impairing carcinogen metabolism, also play a role.

The combination of tobacco use and alcohol consumption is particularly implicated in OSCC.

Betel quid, often containing betel vine leaf, betel (areca) nut, catechu, and slaked lime sometimes with tobacco, appears to be carcinogenic. Some 20% of the world's population use betel. In persons from the developing world, OSCC is seen especially in tobacco or alcohol users and particularly in betel quid users. Various other chewing habits, often containing tobacco, are used in different cultures (eg Qat. Shammah. Toombak).

OTHER FACTORS

Not all tobacco/alcohol users develop cancer, and similarly not all patients with cancer have these habits, and thus other factors must also play a part. These may include:
- Deficiencies of vitamins A, E or C or possibly trace elements
- An impaired ability to metabolise carcinogens which may be hereditory
- An impaired ability to repair DNA damaged by mutagens which may be hereditory
- Immune defects. These may predispose to OSCC, especially lip cancer, which is increased in, eg immunosuppressed organ transplant recipients.

CLINICAL FEATURES

Most oral cancer is carcinoma on the lower lip where it may be preceded by, or associated with, actinic cheilitis (Fig. 2) induced by chronic exposure to sunlight, and typically presents as a swelling or lump (Fig. 3). The other main site is intraorally, especially on the postero-lateral border/ventrum of the tongue (Fig. 4).

Intraoral SCC may present as an indurated lump/ulcer ie a firm infiltration beneath the mucosa (Figs 5-6); a lump sometimes with abnormal supplying blood vessels; a red lesion (erythroplasia); a granular ulcer with fissuring or raised exophytic margins; a white or mixed white and red lesion (Fig. 7); a white lesion (Fig. 8), a non-healing extraction socket; a lesion fixed to deeper tissues or to overlying skin or mucosa; or cervical lymph node enlargement, especially if there is hardness in a lymph node or fixation. SCC should be considered where any of these features persist for more than three weeks (Fig. 9).

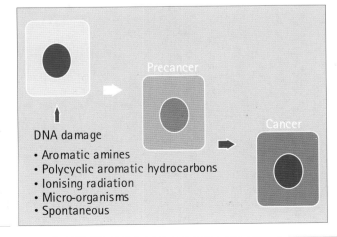

DNA damage
- Aromatic amines
- Polycyclic aromatic hydrocarbons
- Ionising radiation
- Micro-organisms
- Spontaneous

Fig. 1 Carcinogenesis

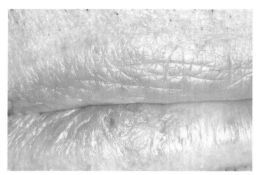

Fig. 2 Actinic keratosis

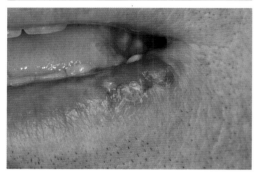

Fig. 3 Early squamous carcinoma of the lip

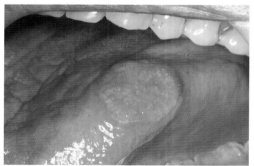

Fig. 4 SCC tongue

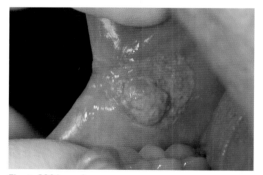

Fig. 5 SCC buccal mucosa

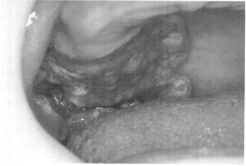

Fig. 6 SCC in soft palate complex

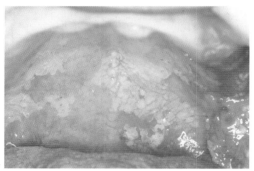

Fig. 7 SCC arising in leukoplakia

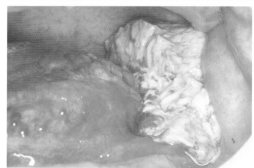

Fig. 8 Squamous cell carcinoma

It is important to note that, in patients with OSCC, a second primary neoplasm may be seen elsewhere in the upper aerodigestive tract in up to 25% over three years. Indeed, many patients treated for OSCC succumb to a second primary

Table 3 TNM classification of malignant neoplasm[a]

Primary tumour size (T)	
Tx	No available information
T0	No evidence of primary tumour
Tis	Only carcinoma in situ
T1, T2, T3, T 4	Increasing size of tumour[b]
Regional lymph node involvement (N)	
Nx	Nodes could not or were not assessed
N0	No clinically positive nodes
N1	Single clinically positive ipsilateral node less than 3 cm in diameter
N2	Single clinically positive ipsilateral node 3 cm to 6 cm in diameter, or multiple clinically positive homolateral nodes, none more than 6 cm in diameter
N2a	Single clinically positive ipsilateral node 3 cm to 6 cm in diameter
N2b	Multiple clinically positive ipsilateral nodes, none more than 6 cm in diameter
N3	Massive ipsilateral node(s), bilateral nodes, or contralateral node(s)
N3a	Clinically positive ipsilateral node(s), one more than 6 cm in diameter
N3b	Bilateral clinically positive nodes
N3c	Contralateral clinically positive node(s)
Involvement by distant metastases(M)	
Mx	Distant metastasis was not assessed
M0	No evidence of distant metastasis
M1, M2, M3	Distant metastasis is present. Increasing degrees of metastatic involvement, including distant nodes

a Several other classifications are available, e.g. STNM (S = site).
b T1 maximum diameter 2 cm; T2 maximum diameter of 4 cm; T3 maximum diameter over 4 cm. T4 massive tumour greater than 4 cm diameter, with involvement of antrum, pterygoid muscles, base of tongue or skin.

Table 4 Prognosis for intraoral carcinoma		
Stage	TNM	Approximate % survival at 5 years
I	T1 N0 M0	85
II	T2 N0 M0	65
III	T3 N0 M0 T1, T2 or T3 N1 M0	40
IV	Any T4,N2,N3 or M1	10

Adapted from Sciubba 2001

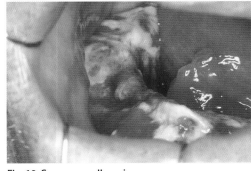
Fig. 10 Squamous cell carcinoma

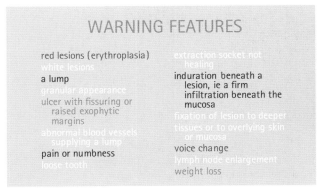

WARNING FEATURES

red lesions (erythroplasia)
white lesions
a lump
granular appearance
ulcer with fissuring or raised exophytic margins
abnormal blood vessels supplying a lump
pain or numbness
loose tooth

extraction socket not healing
induration beneath a lesion, ie a firm infiltration beneath the mucosa
fixation of lesion to deeper tissues or to overlying skin or mucosa
voice change
lymph node enlargement
weight loss

Fig. 9 Warning features suggestive of carcinoma

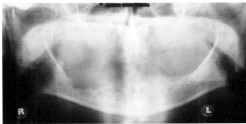
Fig. 11 Radiograph from patient in Fig. 10, showing bony destruction in the mandible

tumour rather than a recurrence of the original tumour.

DIAGNOSIS
Management of early cancers appears to confer survival advantage and is also associated with less morbidity and needs less mutilating surgery. Thus it is important to be suspicious of oral lesions — particularly in patients at high risk, such as older males with habits such as the use of tobacco, alcohol or betel, particularly if there is a history of previous OSCC. There should thus be a high index of suspicion, especially of a solitary lesion. Clinicians should be aware that single ulcers, lumps, red patches, or white patches — particularly if any of these are persisting for more than three weeks, may be manifestations of malignancy.

Frank tumours should be inspected and palpated to determine extent of spread; for tumours in the posterior tongue, examination under general anaesthetic by a specialist may facilitate this.

The whole oral mucosa should be examined as there may be widespread dysplastic mucosa ('field change') or even a second neoplasm. The cervical lymph nodes and rest of the upper aerodigestive tract (mouth, nares, pharynx, larynx, oesophagus) must be examined.

Investigations
It is essential to determine whether bone or muscles are involved or if metastases – initially to regional lymph nodes and later to liver, bone and brain — are present. Imaging may be needed (Figs 10-11). Another important aspect in planning treatment is to determine if there is malignant disease elsewhere, particularly whether other primary tumours are present, and therefore endoscopy may form part of the initial assessment.

Urgent referral should be made and a biopsy by a specialist is preferable but, if a specialist opinion is not readily accessible, an incisional biopsy can be done in general practice if the practitioner is both competent and confident to carry this out. If you are concerned, phone, email or write for an URGENT specialist opinion which is indicated if you feel a diagnosis of cancer is seriously possible or if the diagnosis is unclear.

One of the most difficult clinical situations in which clinicians find themselves is with the patient in whom cancer is suspected. Patient communication and information are important. If the patient is to be referred to a specialist for a diagnosis and insists (rightly) on a full explanation as to why there is a need for a second opinion, it is probably better to say that you are trained more to be suspicious but hope the lesion is nothing to worry about, though you would be failing in your duty if you did not ask for a second opinion. However, you should leave discussion of actual diagnosis, treatment and prognosis to the specialist concerned, as only they are in a position to give accurate facts regarding future management and prognosis to the patient concerned.

The biopsy should be sufficiently large to include enough suspect tissue to give the pathologist a chance to make a diagnosis and not to have to request a further specimen. Since red rather than white areas are most likely to show dysplasia, a biopsy should be taken of the former. Some authorities always take several biopsies at the first visit in order to avoid the delay, anxiety and aggravation resulting from a negative pathology report in a patient who is strongly suspected as suffering from a malignant neoplasm. Attempts to clinically highlight probable dysplastic areas before biopsy, eg by the use of toluidine blue dye and other vital stains, may be of some help where there is widespread 'field change'. Molecular techniques are being introduced for prognostication in potentially malignant lesions and tumours, and to identify nodal metastases.

Finally, the person organising treatment also needs to ensure that the patient is as prepared as possible for the major surgery required, particularly in terms of general anaesthesia, potential blood loss and ability to metabolise drugs, and to address any potential medical, dental or oral problems pre-operatively, to avoid complications. Therefore almost invariably indicated are an assessment of the dentition and periodontum and:

- Medical examination
- Biopsy of equivocal neck lymph nodes
- Jaw and chest radiography
- MRI or CT
- Electrocardiography
- Blood tests.

Selected patients may also need:

- Bronchoscopy – if chest radiography reveals lesions
- Endoscopy – if there is a history of tobacco use
- Gastroscopy – if PEG (per-endoscopic gastrostomy) is to be used for feeding post-surgery
- Liver ultrasound – to exclude metastases
- Doppler duplex flow studies and angiography: to help in planning free flaps for reconstruction.

MANAGEMENT

Cancer treatment is a team approach involving a range of specialties including surgeons, anaesthetists, oncologists, nursing staff, dental staff, nutritionists, speech and physiotherapists, and others. Increasingly, Head and Neck Tumour Boards are being developed along with Cancer Networks to facilitate the collaboration of providers of cancer services to provide seamless care based on best practice (eg http://www.eastman.ucl.ac.uk/hntb/index.html). Consensus guidelines to treatment are now being published.

OSCC is now treated largely by surgery and/or radiotherapy to control the primary tumour and metastases in cervical lymph nodes. Treatment and prognosis are assessed from the TNM classification (Tables 3 and 4).

The planning phase includes discussions regarding restorative and surgical interventions required before cancer treatment, including osseointegrated implants and jaw and occlusal reconstruction. Therapy is also planned to avoid post-operative complications. As much oral care as possible should be completed before starting cancer treatment.

Oral care is especially important when radiotherapy is to be given, since there is a liability particularly to mucositis, xerostomia and other complications, and a risk of osteonecrosis – the initiating factor for which is often trauma, such as tooth extraction, or ulceration from an appliance, or oral infection.

Websites and patient information
http://www.entnet.org/cancer.html
http://cancer.med.upenn.edu/new/index.html
http://www.oralcancer.org
http://www.nlm.nih.gov/medlineplus/oralcancer.html
http://www.dh.gov.uk/PolicyAndGuidance/HealthAndSocialCareTopics/Cancer/fs/en
http://www.mayoclinic.com/invoke.cfm?objec-tid=F4D66AB7-A46B-46EF-BC71F844B12232A0
http://www.rdoc.org.uk/

Patients to refer
All patients with suspected oral malignancy

Patients with erythroplasia

Patients with other potentially malignant lesions

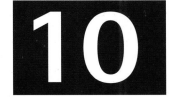

- Orofacial pain usually has a local cause.
- Dental caries and sequelae are the main causes.
- A careful history is crucial to the diagnosis.
- Lancinating pain is typical of trigeminal neuralgia.
- Chronic pain in the absence of organic causes, may be psychogenic.

Orofacial pain

PAIN

Pain in the teeth, mouth, face or head usually has a local cause, often the sequelae of dental caries (odontogenic pain). However, psychogenic, neurological and vascular conditions, and conditions where pain is referred from elsewhere, may be responsible (Table 1).

Dental staff will be well versed in pain of local causes and therefore this article discusses mainly the conditions in which specialist help may be indicated. Many of the conditions discussed in previous articles in this series may cause pain.

The real significance to the patient of orofacial pain apart from the pain itself, can range from the benign to potentially lethal conditions. Some orofacial pain or headaches have an obvious but relatively unimportant cause (eg a hangover – caused mainly by the acetaldehyde resulting from metabolism of alcohol or headaches from glyceryl trinitrate); others types of pain have no obvious underlying organic pathology (and are thus termed medically unexplained symptoms [MUS], eg atypical facial pain). Some can threaten important faculties such as sight (eg giant cell arteritis), or even life (eg brain tumours).

DIAGNOSIS OF OROFACIAL PAIN

The history is by far the most important means of diagnosing orofacial pain (Fig. 1).

In order to differentiate the widely disparate causes, it is essential to determine key points about the pain, especially:
- **Location.** Valuable information can be

obtained by asking if the pain is localised or diffuse, and watching the patient's reaction.

Table 1 Causes of orofacial pain

Local disorders
- Teeth and supporting tissues
- Jaws
- Maxillary antrum and nares
- Salivary glands
- Pharynx
- Eyes

Neurological disorders
- Idiopathic trigeminal neuralgia
- Malignant neoplasms involving the trigeminal nerve
- Glossopharyngeal neuralgia
- Herpes zoster (including post-herpetic neuralgia)
- Multiple sclerosis

Possible psychogenic causes
- Atypical facial pain
- Burning mouth syndrome
- Temporomandibular pain-dysfunction

Vascular disorders
- Migraine
- Migrainous neuralgia
- Giant cell arteritis

Referred pain
- Aural
- Cardiorespiratory
    Angina
- Lesions in the neck or chest (including lung cancer)

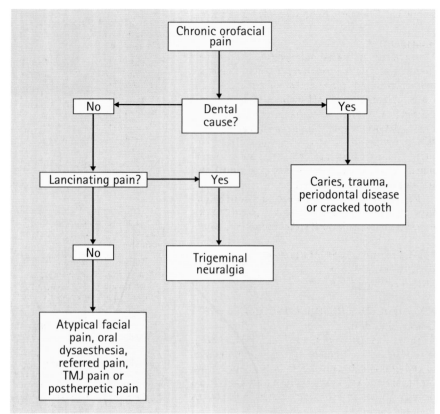

Fig.1 Chronic orofacial pain

For example, patients frequently point with one finger when describing pain of dental causes or trigeminal neuralgia, but atypical facial pain is much more diffuse, and may radiate across the midline.

- **Character.** Patients should be asked about the severity and character of the pain ie whether the pain is 'sharp', 'dull', 'aching', 'throbbing' or 'shooting'. However, bear in mind that patients often have difficulty finding adequate descriptors. Ask the patient to rate the pain severity on a scale of zero (no pain) to 10 (most severe pain that the patient has experienced), or ask them to mark this on a line divided into 10 equal sections (visual analogue scale) or use an assessment instrument such as the McGill Pain Questionnaire. These 'tools' help assess the severity of pain, accepting always that it is subjective, and they may also be useful in monitoring the response to treatment. Disturbance of the normal sleep pattern by pain is also useful in assessing the severity.
- **Duration.** The average duration of each episode may help diagnosis. For example, pain from exposed dentine is fairly transient (lasting only for seconds) while the pain from pulpitis lasts for a much longer period. Trigeminal neuralgia is a brief lancinating pain lasting up to about five seconds, although some patients report a persistent background less severe pain – more of a dull ache; migrainous neuralgia typically lasts 30 to 45 minutes, while atypical facial pain is typically dull and persistent.
- **Frequency and periodicity.** Determine whether the pain occurs at specific times or related to specific events. A 'pain diary' can help. For example, the pain of temporo-

mandibular pain dysfunction syndrome may be more severe on waking if this is associated with nocturnal parafunctional activity such as clenching or tooth grinding. The pain from obstructive sialadenitis is related to meals. The pain of sinusitis is often aggravated by lying down. Periodic migrainous neuralgia frequently disturbs the patient's sleep at a specific time each night, around 2am. One patient seen by the authors complained of pain fairly typical of periodic migrainous neuralgia, yet appearing around 2pm; it turned out he was a long-distance night driver, sleeping mainly during the day!

- **Precipitating, aggravating and relieving factors.** It may be necessary to resort to leading questions to ask if temperature, biting, posture, analgesics, alcohol etc affect the pain. For example, heat often aggravates dental pain; touching a trigger zone may precipitate trigeminal neuralgia attacks, stress may worsen atypical facial pain, and alcohol may induce episodes of migrainous neuralgia.
- **Associated features.** Some types of pain may be associated with other features which are helpful diagnostically, such as the swollen face in dental abscess, nausea and vomiting in migraine, or nasal stuffiness or lacrimation in migrainous neuralgia.

The cause of most orofacial pain is established mainly from the history, and examination findings are also helpful, not least in excluding local pathology. However, it is important to consider the usefulness of a specialist who can arrange additional investigations, particularly imaging of the head and neck, using CT or MRI or ultra-sound. It is crucial not to miss detecting organic disease and thus mislabelling the patient as having psychogenic pain, and not to miss a brain tumour underlying a patient with supposed 'idiopathic' trigeminal neuralgia.

LOCAL CAUSES OF OROFACIAL PAIN
Odontogenic pain
Most orofacial pain is related to dental disease – odontogenic causes - and will not be described further.

Mucosal pain
Pain from oral mucosal lesions can be either localised or diffuse. Localised pain is usually associated with a mucosal break, either an erosion (a partial thickness loss of epithelium) or ulcer (a full thickness loss of epithelium). Of course, the distinction between these painful conditions can at times be difficult or impossible and many patients have both.

Diffuse pain may also be caused by infection, or a systemic underlying deficiency state or other factors, and is usually then described as 'soreness' or sometimes 'burning'.

Mucosal pain may be aggravated by sour, acidic, spicy, or salty foods, so that few affected patients can tolerate or enjoy citrus fruits or tomatoes for example. The area is usually also tender to touch.

Other local causes of orofacial pain

Pain from the jaws can be caused by infection, direct trauma, malignancies, and rarely by Paget's disease. However, unless associated with infection or jaw fracture, retained roots and impacted teeth, and lesions such as cysts, are usually painless.

Malignant tumours usually produce deep, boring pain, sometimes associated with paraesthesia or anaesthesia but odontogenic and other benign tumours of the bone do not normally produce pain. Lip numbness or tingling, therefore, may herald a tumour in the jaw bone.

Pain from salivary gland disorders is mainly caused by duct obstruction, sometimes by infection or a tumour. The pain is usually localised to the affected gland, may be quite severe, and may be intensified by increased saliva production such as before and with meals. Examination may reveal a swollen salivary gland sometimes with tenderness and/or a degree of trismus.

Diseases of the paranasal sinuses and nasopharynx which can cause oral and/or facial pain include sinusitis and tumours – which can remain undetected until they have reached an advanced stage. Any suggestion of a discharge from the nose, or obstruction to breathing, cheek swelling or numbness or tingling of the lip should be taken seriously as such structures may herald an antral carcinoma.

On occasions if there is dehiscence of the mental nerve, as a result of resorption of the alveolar ridge, pain is caused by pressure from a denture.

TEMPOROMANDIBULAR JOINT PAIN

Pain from the TMJ may result from dysfunction, trauma, inflammation, and very rarely tumours – either in the head and neck, or even lungs.

Temporomandibular pain–dysfunction syndrome

Temporomandibular pain-dysfunction syndrome is a very common problem, characterised by pain, clicking and jaw locking or limitation of movements of the jaw. Afflicting young women mainly, factors which have been implicated include over-opening of the mouth, muscle overactivity (eg bruxism, clenching), TMJ disruption and psychiatric history (eg anxiety, stressful life events). Precipitating factors may include local trauma, wide mouth opening, or emotional upset.

Diagnosis

Diagnosis is clinical. Pain from TMJ disease is usually dull, poorly localised, may radiate widely, is usually intensified by movement of the mandible and may be associated with trismus because of spasm in the masticatory muscles.

Examination may reveal a click from the joint, limited jaw movements, and tender masticatory muscles. Any suggestion of a

swollen and/or warm joint, suggests true arthritis.

Management

Most patients recover spontaneously and progression to arthritis is virtually unknown. Therefore reassurance and conservative measures are the main management. TMJ pain-dysfunction can usually be effectively managed in general practice.

Practitioners are usually well versed with this problem but possible options for treatment in a primary care environment are summarised in the Key points box (see right) and patient guidance in Table 2.

Recalcitrant cases may need specialist attention and may warrant anxiolytics or antidepressants, particularly if simple measures fail.

Websites and patient information

http://www.aaop.org
http://www.tmjd.com/

NEUROLOGICAL (NEUROPATHIC) CAUSES OF OROFACIAL PAIN

Sensory innervation of the mouth, face and scalp depends on the trigeminal nerve, so that diseases affecting this nerve anywhere in the course from orofacial region to brain, can cause orofacial pain or indeed sensory loss – sometimes with serious implications.

Key points for dentists: Management of TMJ pain–dysfunction

- Reassurance/explanation of the benign and self-limiting nature of the problem
- Rest (eg soft diet and limitation of movement)
- Anti-inflammatory analgesic (eg ibuprofen 400 mg three times a day)
- Occlusal splint therapy
- Local physiotherapy

Key points for patients: Temporomandibular (TMJ) pain–dysfunction

- This is a common condition
- It appears to be related to stress, joint damage or habits involving the teeth and joints (eg tooth clenching or grinding)
- There are no serious long-term consequences; arthritis does not result
- The symptoms usually clear spontaneously after some months but meantime, rest, exercises, splints, or drugs may help.

Table 2 Steps to manage TMJ pain dysfunction

Rest yourself and your jaw

Relax and practice stress reduction

Exercise regularly

Eat soft foods and avoid hard, crusty foods like nuts or hard bread or those that need chewing a great deal

Chew on your back teeth, not the front ones

Eat small bites

Sleep on your side

Avoid joint or muscle damage by avoiding:

- contact sports; wear a mouthguard if you must play contact sports
- excessive jaw use in yawning, grinding and clenching
- chewing gum
- habits such as biting finger nails, pens and pencils or lip
- excessive mouth-opening in long dental appointments
- general anaesthesia
- cradling the telephone between head and shoulder
- wind instrument playing

Reduce muscle pain with analgesics and by applying:

- cold packs for 10 minutes every three hours for 72 hours after injury
- hot packs for 20 minutes every three hours to uninjured joints/muscles

Re-educate the jaw opening:

Open your mouth with a hinge movement: exercise your jaw twice daily, opening five times in front of a mirror, ensuring the jaw opens vertically downwards without deviating sideways

Exercise your jaw three times daily for five timed minutes:

- close your mouth on the back teeth
- put the tip of your tongue on the palate behind your front teeth
- move the tongue back across the palate as far as it will go
- keep the tongue in this position with the teeth closed for 10 seconds
- open your mouth slowly until the tongue starts to leave the palate
- keep that position for 10 seconds
- close your mouth
- repeat over five minutes

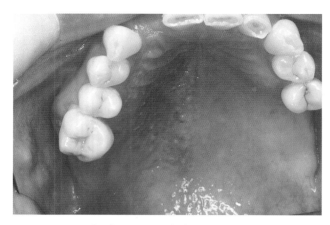

Fig. 2 Herpes zoster, palate

Such causes include:

- trauma
- cerebrovascular disease
- demyelinating disease (eg multiple sclerosis)
- neoplasia (eg nasopharyngeal, antral or brain tumours); (or infections such as herpes zoster or HIV/AIDS (Fig. 2).

Idiopathic trigeminal neuralgia

Idiopathic trigeminal neuralgia (ITN) is an uncommon nerve disorder that causes episodes of unilateral intense, stabbing, electric shock-like pain in the areas of the face where the branches of the nerve are distributed – lips, eyes, nose, scalp, forehead, upper jaw, or lower jaw. ITN onset is mainly in the 50-70 year age group.

The cause of ITN is unclear, but one hypothesis is that a cerebral blood vessel becomes atherosclerotic and therefore less flexible with age, then pressing on the roots of the trigeminal nerve in the posterior cranial fossa – causing neuronal discharge.

The characteristic features of ITN are summarised as:

- Paroxysmal attacks of facial or frontal pain which lasts a few seconds to less than two minutes. These attacks occur especially in the morning, and rarely cause sleep disturbance.
- Pain has at least four of the following characteristics:
  - Distribution along one or more division of the trigeminal nerve.
  - Sudden intense, sharp superficial, stabbing or burning in quality.
  - Pain intensity severe.
  - Precipitation from trigger areas or by certain daily activities such as eating, talking, washing the face, shaving, or cleaning the teeth.
  - Between paroxysms, the patient is usually entirely asymptomatic. Some patients experience a dull ache at other times.
- No neurological deficit.
- Attacks are stereotyped in the individual patient.
- Exclusion of other causes of facial pain by history, physical examination and special investigations when necessary.

A less common form of the disorder called 'Atypical Trigeminal Neuralgia' may cause less intense, constant, dull burning or aching pain, sometimes with occasional electric shock-like stabs. Both forms of the disorder most often affect one side of the face, but some patients experience pain at different times on both sides.

Diagnosis

ITN is universally considered to be one of the most painful afflictions known. Severe pain suggestive of ITN but with physical signs such as facial sensory or motor impairment can result from lesions discussed above. These serious conditions must therefore be excluded by history, examination; including neurological assessment especially of cranial nerves, and investigations; including imaging (usually MRI) to exclude space-occupying or demyelinating disease, and blood tests to exclude infections and systemic vasculitides.

Only then can the term *idiopathic* (benign) trigeminal neuralgia be used.

Management

Few patients with ITN have spontaneous remission and thus treatment is usually indicated. However, ITN is often an intermittent disease with apparent remissions lasting months or years but recurrence is common and very often the pain spreads to involve a wider area over time and the intervals between episodes tend to shorten.

Patients with supposed ITN are best seen at an early stage by a Specialist in order to confirm the diagnosis and initiate treatment. In the acute situation the patient's symptoms may be controlled on a short term basis with injection of a regional local anaesthetic.

Medical treatment, typically using anticonvulsants, is successful for most patients (Table 3). Carbamazepine is the main drug used, but it is not an analgesic and must be given continuously prophylactically for long periods, and under strict medical surveillance. Adverse effects must be monitored, including:

- balance (disturbed – ataxia); this tends to be the feature that limits the dose of carbamazepine
- blood pressure (may increase); patients must have a baseline test and then blood pressure estimations for three months, then six-monthly
- blood tests – mainly for liver function (may become impaired); and bone marrow function (red and white cells and/or platelets may be depressed).

Table 3 Medical and surgical treatments for ITN

Medical

Carbamazepine
Gabapentin
Phenytoin
Lamotrigine
Baclofen

Surgical

Cryotherapy
Balloon compression of trigeminal ganglion
Microvascular decompression
Gamma knife surgery

Other agents such as gabapentin, phenytoin, lamotrigine and baclofen are available and some patients also report having reduced or relieved pain by means of alternative medical therapies such as acupuncture, chiropractic adjustment, self-hypnosis or meditation.

Should medical care become ineffective, or produce excessive undesirable side effects, neurosurgical procedures are available to relieve pressure on the nerve or to reduce nerve sensitivity.

Websites and patient information
http://www.painfoundation.org/
http://www.tna-support.org/
http://www.mayoclinic.com

GLOSSOPHARYNGEAL NEURALGIA
Glossopharyngeal neuralgia is much less common than trigeminal neuralgia. Occasionally glossopharyngeal neuralgia is secondary to tumours. The pain is of a similar nature but affects the throat and ear, and typically is triggered by swallowing or coughing. Carbamazepine is usually less effective than for trigeminal neuralgia and adequate relief of pain can be difficult. A specialist opinion is warranted to investigate and manage these patients.

HERPETIC AND POST-HERPETIC NEURALGIA
Herpes zoster (shingles), the recrudescence of herpes-varicella-zoster virus latent in sensory ganglia after chickenpox, is often preceded and accompanied by neuralgia, but a unilateral rash and ulceration is typical (Fig. 2). Neuralgia may also persist (post-herpetic neuralgia) after the rash has resolved and can cause continuous burning pain, in contrast to the lancinating pain of trigeminal neuralgia, which also affects mainly elderly patients. A specialist opinion is warranted to investigate and manage these patients.

PSYCHOGENIC CAUSES OF OROFACIAL PAIN
Psychogenic (tension) headaches caused by anxiety or stress-induced muscle tension are common, especially in young adults. The pain typically, affects the frontal, occipital and/or temporal regions, as a constant ache or bandlike pressure, often worse by the evening, but usually abates with rest. Similar problems can affect the orofacial region.

Reassurance may be effective but the pain may also be helped by massage, warmth, by non-steroidal anti-inflammatory drugs (NSAIDs), or by benzodiazepines — which are both anxiolytic and mild muscle relaxants, or by complementary therapies.

In some studies, nearly 40% of the population have reported frequent headaches and orofacial pain. The reason behind conditions with a psychogenic component, sometimes termed medically unexplained symptoms (MUS), may include:
- Possible links between neuro-humoural mechanisms and altered CNS function.
- The heightening of bodily sensations (lowered pain threshold) as a consequence of physiological processes such as autonomic arousal, muscle tension, hyperventilation, or inactivity.
- Misattribution of normal sensations to serious physical disorders.

Features common to most MUS include:
- Constant chronic discomfort or pain.
- Pain often of a dull boring or burning type.
- Pain poorly localised.
- Pain may cross the midline to involve the other side or may move elsewhere.
- Pain which rarely wakens the patient from sleep.
- Total lack of objective signs of organic disease.
- All investigations to identify an underlying organic illness are also negative.
- There are often recent adverse 'life events' such as bereavement or family illness.
- There are often multiple oral and/or other MUS, such as headaches, chronic back or neck pain, pruritus, irritable bowel syndrome, insomnia, numbness or dysmenorrhoea.
- Cure is uncommon in most, yet few sufferers seem to try or persist using analgesics.

Patients may bring diaries of their symptoms to emphasise their problem. Some have termed this the 'malady of small bits of paper' and though there is by no means always a psychogenic basis, such notes characterise patients with MUS. These days, this is being replaced by Internet print-outs, which are also increasingly brought by well-informed patients who have no psychogenic problems whatsoever.

Occasional patients quite deliberately induce painful oral lesions and some have Munchausen's syndrome, where they behave in such a fashion as to appear to want operative intervention.

The most common types of orofacial pain with a strong psychogenic component are:
- atypical facial pain
- oral dysaesthesia (burning mouth syndrome: BMS)
- atypical odontalgia
- the syndrome of oral complaints
- some clinicians also include temporomandibular pain-dysfunction in this category.

ATYPICAL FACIAL PAIN
Atypical facial pain (AFP) is a constant chronic orofacial discomfort or pain, defined by the International Headache Society as facial pain not fulfilling other criteria. Therefore, like burning mouth syndrome (see below), it is also a diagnosis reached only by the exclusion of organic disease; there are no physical signs, investigations are all negative and it is an MUS. Atypical facial pain is fairly common, affecting probably around 1-2% of the population. It is sometimes termed persistent idiopathic facial pain.

ORAL MEDICINE

Atypical facial pain is often of a dull boring or burning type character and ill-defined location and there is:
- a total lack of objective signs
- a negative result from all investigations
- no clear explanation as to cause
- poor response to treatment.

Patients are often middle-aged or older and 70% or more are females. Most sufferers from AFP are otherwise normal individuals who are or have been, under extreme stress such as bereavement, or concern about cancer. There are often recent adverse life-events, such as bereavement or family illness and/or dental or oral interventive procedures.

Clinical features
History findings in AFP include pain mainly in the upper jaw, of distribution unrelated to the anatomical distribution of the trigeminal nerve, poorly localised, and sometimes crossing the midline to involve the other side or moving to another site. Pain is often of a deep, dull boring or burning, chronic discomfort, and persists for most or all of the day but does not waken the patient from sleep. However the patient may report difficulty sleeping.

There may also be multiple oral and/or other psychogenic related complaints, such as dry mouth, bad or altered taste, thirst, headaches, chronic back pain, irritable bowel syndrome or dysmenorrhoea. Patients only uncommonly use analgesics to try and control the pain but there is a high level of use of health care services. There have often already been multiple (unsatisfactory) consultations and attempts at treatment.

Pain is accompanied by altered behaviour, anxiety or depression. Over 50% of such patients are depressed or hypochondriacal, and some have lost or been separated from parents in childhood. Many lack insight and will persist in blaming organic diseases (or health care professionals) for their pain.

Clinical examination is unremarkable with a total lack of objective physical (including neurological) signs. All imaging studies and blood investigations are negative.

Diagnosis of AFP
Diagnosis of atypical facial pain is clinical through careful examination of the mouth, perioral structures, and cranial nerves, and imaging (tooth/jaw/sinus radiography and MRI/CT scan) to exclude organic disease such as space-occupying or demyelinating diseases (Table 4).

MANAGEMENT OF PATIENTS SUFFERING ATYPICAL FACIAL PAIN OR PAIN WITH A PSYCHOGENIC BASIS
Few patients with AFP have spontaneous remission and thus treatment is usually indicated (Fig. 3).

Reassurance and attention to any factors such as the dentures or haematinic deficiencies

may be indicated, but active dental or oral surgical treatment, or attempts at 'hormone replacement', or polypharmacy in the absence of any specific indication, should be avoided. Do not repeat examinations or investigations at subsequent appointments, since this only serves to reinforce abnormal illness behaviour and health fears.

Avoid attempts at relieving pain by operative intervention – since these are rarely successful; indeed, active dental measures such as restorative treatment, endodontics or oral surgical treatment, in the absence of any specific indication, should be avoided as they may simply reinforce the patient's perception that the pain has an organic basis.

However, it is important where possible, to identify and relieve factors which lower the pain threshold (fatigue, anxiety and depression). Simple analgesics such as NSAIDs should be tried initially, before embarking on more potent preparations.

Patient information is a very important aspect in management. Cognitive-behavioural therapy (CBT) or a specialist referral may be indicated.

It is important to clearly acknowledge the reality of the patient's symptoms and distress and never attempt to trivialise or dismiss them.

Try to explain the psychosomatic background to the problem, ascribing the symptoms to causes for which the patient cannot be blamed

Set goals which include helping the patient cope with the symptoms rather than attempting any impossible cure

Offer referral to a specialist or a trial of antidepressants, explaining that these agents are being used to treat the symptoms not depression, that some antidepressants have analgesic activity and that antidepressants have been shown in controlled trials to be effective for this problem, even in non-depressed persons.

Websites and patient information
http://facial-neuralgia.org/conditions/atfp.html

BURNING MOUTH 'SYNDROME' (BMS)
There may be definable organic causes of this type of complaint, often described as a burning sensation (Table 5), and a patient in such pain may well also manifest psychological reactions to the experience. However, burning mouth 'syndrome' (BMS; also known as glossopyrosis; glossodynia; oral dysaesthesia; or stomatodynia) is the term usually used when symptoms described as a burning sensation, exist in the absence of identifiable organic aetiological factors. BMS is often a MUS but it must also be recognised that it may well not be a single entity.

BMS is a fairly common chronic complaint, affecting up to 2.6 % of the population and seen especially in middle aged or elderly patients, particularly in females, in a ratio of more than 3:1 and even as high as 7:1. There is no specific relationship to hormonal changes, despite the fact that BMS is often seen in middle aged or elderly peri- or post-menopausal females. BMS has been reported in 10-40% of women presenting for treatment of menopausal symptoms.

Defined clinical conditions that must be excluded since they can also present with burning include:
- erythema migrans (geographic tongue)
- lichen planus
- dry mouth (xerostomia)
- candidosis
- glossitis such as may be associated with haematinic (iron, folic acid, vitamin B) deficiency
- diabetes.

Uncommon causes that may need to be considered include:
- hypothyroidism
- lupus erythematosus
- mucositis
- drugs (especially angiotensin-converting enzyme [ACE] inhibitors; protease inhibitors; cytotoxic agents; clonazepam)
- hypersensitivity (to sodium metabisulphite, nuts, dental materials and other substances)
- galvanic reactions to metals in the mouth.

Organic problems which sometimes present with no detectable clinical lesions, but that can cause similar symptoms include:
- A haematological deficiency state (deficiencies in iron, folic acid or vitamin B).
- Restricted tongue space from poor denture construction.
- Parafunction such as nocturnal bruxism or tongue-thrusting.
- Neuropathy – such as follows damage to the chorda tympani nerve.

No precipitating cause for BMS can be identified in over 50% of the patients but, in others, a psychogenic cause such as anxiety, depression or cancerophobia can be identified in about 20%, and in some patients, BMS may be due to a neuropathy or appears to follow either dental intervention or an upper respiratory tract infection.

Clinical features

BMS most frequently affects the tongue, but it can also affect the palate or, less commonly, the lips or lower alveolus. The history is that the burning sensation is chronic, usually bilateral, often relieved by eating and drinking, in contrast to pain caused by organic lesions which is typically aggravated by eating. Alcohol may also relieve or reduce the symptoms.

Patients with BMS often have multiple oral and/or other psychogenic related complaints, such as dry mouth, bad or altered taste, thirst, headaches, chronic back pain, irritable bowel syndrome or dysmenorrhoea. There may be changes in sleep patterns and mood and, though patients only uncommonly use analgesics to try and control the symptoms, there

have often already been multiple consultations. Interestingly, patients with BMS also have heightened ability to taste – they are 'supertasters'.

Examination shows no clinically detectable signs of mucosal disease or tenderness or swelling of the tongue or affected area, and no neurological or other objective signs.

Diagnosis

Diagnosis of BMS is clinical and it is important to exclude the organic causes outlined above. Importantly, all investigations prove normal.

Investigations indicated, may include:
- laboratory screening for anaemia, a vitamin or iron deficiency (blood tests)
- diabetes (blood and urine analyses)
- thyroid dysfunction (blood analyses)
- xerostomia (salivary flow rates)
- candidosis (oral rinse).
- psychological screening using, for example, the Hospital Anxiety and Depression (HAD) scale.

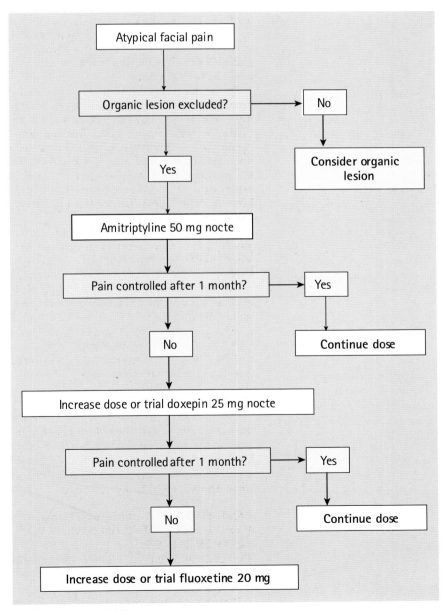

Fig. 3 Management of AFP

Table 4 Differentiation of important types of chronic orofacial pain

	Idiopathic trigeminal neuralgia	Atypical facial pain	Migrainous neuralgia
Age (years)	>50	30-50	30-50
Gender	F>M	F>M	M>F
Site	Unilateral, mandible or maxilla	+ Bilateral, maxilla	Retro-orbital
Associated features	-	+/- Depression	+/- Conjunctival injection +/- Lacrimation +/- Nasal congestion
Character	Lancinating	Dull	Boring
Duration of episodes	Brief (seconds)	Continual	Few hours
Usual timing of pain	Daytime	Daytime	Night time
Precipitating factors	Trigger areas	+/- adverse life events	+/- Alcohol
Main treatments	Carbamazepine	Cognitive behavioural therapy, antidepressants	Oxygen, sumatriptan

Management is as discussed above for AFP.

Websites and patient information
http://www.mssm.edu/msjournal/65/05_miy.pdf
http://www.go4hope.org
http://www.mayoclinic.com

ATYPICAL ODONTALGIA
Atypical odontalgia is pain and hypersensitive teeth in the absence of detectable pathology. The pain is typically indistinguishable from pulpitis or periodontitis but is aggravated by dental intervention. Probably a variant of atypical facial pain, it should be managed similarly.

The syndrome of oral complaints
Multiple pains and other complaints may occur simultaneously or sequentially, and relief is rarely found (or admitted). may bring diaries of their symptoms to emphasise their problem.

VASCULAR CAUSES OF OROFACIAL PAIN
Several disorders in which the most obvious organic feature is vascular dilatation or constriction can cause orofacial pain. The pain is usually obviously in the face or head rather than in the mouth alone but occasionally can involve both, and can be difficult to differentiate from other causes of orofacial pain. These disorders include:
- Migraine (usually obvious and not causing oral pain alone, and therefore not included here).
- Migrainous neuralgia.
- Giant cell arteritis.
- Migrainous neuralgia (cluster headache).

Migrainous neuralgia is less common than migraine but more likely to cause orofacial pain. Males are mainly affected and attacks often begin about middle age (Table 5). The pain is unilateral, occurs in attacks, is burning and 'boring' in character, and localised around the eye usually. Generally, the attacks commence , and often awaken the patient, at the same time each night or in the early hours of the morning – hence the term 'alarm clock headache'. This pain may be associated with profuse watering and 'congestion' of the conjunctiva, rhinorrhoea and nasal obstruction on the affected side. The attacks usually end in less than one hour. Attacks are sometimes precipitated by alcohol.

Migrainous neuralgia is managed by a specialist, with a variety of agents, including sumatriptan, beta-blockers, indometacin, or with oxygen inhalations.

CRANIAL ARTERITIS (TEMPORAL ARTERITIS; GIANT-CELL ARTERITIS)
Cranial arteritis is a febrile disease, in which giant cells appear in the arteries and cause a deranged internal elastic lamina. It most commonly affects the elderly.

The headache is intense, deep and aching, throbbing in nature and persistent. It is frequently made worse when the patient lies flat in bed and it may be exacerbated or reduced by digital pressure on the artery involved. Occasionally the artery (usually the superficial temporal artery) may be enlarged and tender. It is also characterised by malaise, weakness, weight loss, anorexia, fever, and sweating.

Diagnosis is supported by a raised erythrocyte sedimentation rate (or plasma viscosity). Arterial biopsy demonstrates fragmentation of the internal elastic lamina.

Although it is a self-limiting disease, patients with cranial arteritis may be threatened with loss of vision, and therefore need urgent diagnosis and treatment by a specialist: a systemic corticosteroid (prednisolone) is indicated.

REFERRED CAUSES OF OROFACIAL PAIN
Pain may occasionally be referred to the mouth, face or jaws from the:
- Neck: cervical vertebral disease, especially cervical spondylosis, very occasionally causes pain referred to the face.
- Heart in patients with angina. The pain usually affects the mandible, is initiated by exercise

---

Keypoints for dentists: Burning mouth syndrome

Similar symptoms may be seen in some organic conditions

Blood tests may be required

Psychological assessment can be helpful

Keypoints for patients: Burning mouth syndrome

This is a common condition

The cause is not usually known

It may be a nerve hypersensitivity

It is not infectious

It may occasionally be caused by some mouth conditions, dry mouth, deficiencies, diabetes or drugs

It has no long-term consequences

Blood tests or biopsy may be required

It may be controlled by psychological care or some nerve-calming drugs

---

Table 5 Causes of a burning sensation in the mouth

Local causes

Erythema migrans (geographical tongue)
Lichen planus
Candidosis

Denture problems

Parafunctional activity (eg tongue thrusting habit, clenching)

Systemic causes

Psychogenic
Cancerophobia
Depression
Anxiety states
Hypochondriasis
Deficiency of: Vitamin B, especially B12; Folate; Iron

Dry mouth

Diabetes

Drugs

(especially in the cold) and abates quickly on rest.

- Lungs: orofacial pain emanating from lung cancer is a well-recognised entity and can mimic for example, TMJ pain-dysfunction syndrome.
- Oesophagus; pain plus sialorrhoea may result from oesophageal lesions.
- Styloid process; Eagle's syndrome, a rare disorder due to an elongated styloid process (stylalgia), may cause pain on chewing, swallowing or turning the head.
- Eyes: pain from the eyes, arising for example, from disorders of refraction, retrobulbar neuritis (eg in multiple sclerosis), or glaucoma, can radiate to the orbit, maxilla or frontal region.
- Ears: middle ear disease may cause headaches or pain in the TMJ region. Conversely, oral disease not infrequently causes pain referred to the ear, particularly from lesions of the posterior tongue.
- Pharynx; carcinoma of the pharynx may cause orofacial pain.

A specialist opinion is warranted to investigate and manage these patients.

Patients to refer

Patients with neurological or vascular pain

Trigeminal neuralgia in view of possibility of demyelination or space occupying lesion

Giant cell arteritis in view of risk of blindness

Patients with atypical facial pain who need psychological help

Malignancy

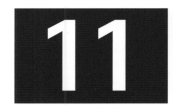

Human immunodeficiency virus infection

Human immunodeficiency viruses (HIV-1 and HIV-2) are RNA retroviruses spread by sexual contact, by sharing needles and/or syringes or, less commonly, through infected blood or blood products transplants. Most HIV transmission worldwide is via heterosexual intercourse, though anal intercourse is more risky than vaginal. Babies born to HIV-infected women may be infected *in utero*, at the time of birth, or may be infected through breast-feeding. Health care professionals have been infected with HIV after sustaining needlestick injuries contaminated with HIV-infected blood or, less frequently, after infected blood has entered an open cut or a mucous membrane (eg the eyes or nose). However, on a global scale, occupational transmission of HIV infection is uncommon. Transmission routes are summarised in Table 1.

Infection with HIV produces HIV infection which eventually results in immunodeficiency and the onset of diseases, at which time the condition is termed HIV disease. When the immune defect produced by HIV becomes so severe that the patient manifests severe opportunistic infections and/or tumours, the condition is known as Acquired Immune Deficiency Syndrome (AIDS) (Fig. 1). The definition of AIDS has changed over the years and now includes parameters such as a CD4 T lymphocyte count below 200 per mm^3, oropharyngeal candidosis, Kaposi's sarcoma and lymphoma.

The Centers for Disease Control and Prevention (CDC) in USA have produced a classification shown in Table 2.

CLINICAL FEATURES

Infection with HIV damages mainly T helper lymphocytes known as CD4 cells. The CD4 cell count falls (with a falling ratio of CD4/CD8 cells). T cell-mediated immune protection thus diminishes, there is generalised lymphadenopathy and patients become predisposed to infection with yeasts and fungi, viruses and mycobacteria.

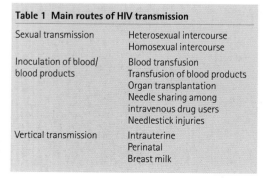

Table 1 Main routes of HIV transmission	
Sexual transmission	Heterosexual intercourse
	Homosexual intercourse
Inoculation of blood/ blood products	Blood transfusion
	Transfusion of blood products
	Organ transplantation
	Needle sharing among intravenous drug users
	Needlestick injuries
Vertical transmission	Intrauterine
	Perinatal
	Breast milk

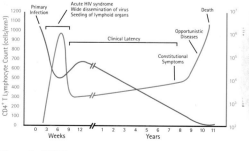

Figure 1. HIV time course

Table 2 CDC classification of HIV and AIDS

	A acute HIV infection	B symptomatic HIV infection, not AIDS	C AIDS
CD4 count/ mm3			
1 = >500	A1	B1	C1
2 = 200-499	A2	B2	C2
3 = <200	A3	B3	C3

		B	C
		Fatigue	**Opportunistic infections**
		Fever	Disseminated cytomegalovirus
		Malaise	Chronic disseminated Herpes simplex
		Weight loss	Progressive multifocal
		Diarrhoea	leucoencephalopathy
		Lymphadenopathy	Tuberculosis
		Wasting	Atypical mycobacterioses
		Oral candidosis	Pneumocystis carinii pneumonia
		Oral hairy leukoplakia	Candidosis of oesophagus, bronchi or
		Herpes zoster	lung
		Immune thrombocytopenia	Chronic cryptosporidiosis
		Perianal herpes	Toxoplasmosis of brain
		Splenomegaly	Isosporiasis
			Disseminated histoplasmosis
			Disseminated coccidioidomycosis
			Cryptococcosis
			Strongyloidiasis extraintestinally.
			Secondary neoplasms
			Kaposi's sarcoma
			Lymphoma: primary of brain
			Non-Hodgkin's lymphoma

The infections that result depend not only on the host immune competence but also on the micro-organisms to which the person is exposed.

Some of these organisms are commensal, such as Candida and some herpesviruses. These may become opportunistic pathogens in the HIV-infected person. The most important infections are fungal such as candidosis and viral such as herpes simplex and cytomegalovirus. *Candida albicans* is the most common pathogen but *Candida krusei*, *Candida glabrata* and *Candida tropicalis* may be seen; new species such as *Candida dubliniensis* have appeared; and antifungal resistance has increased. Herpes simplex infections may become resistant to aciclovir, necessitating the use of other antiviral agents

(eg cidofovir). Herpes zoster may be seen in HIV disease.

Exogenous pathogens such as tuberculous mycobacteria may cause serious disease. Tuberculosis is increasing worldwide, especially in HIV-infected persons in whom it may involve mycobacteria resistant to a range of anti-tubercular drugs (multi-drug resistance; MDR). Exogenous infections also include fungi, parasites such as toxoplasmosis, and *Pneumocystis carinii* pneumonia.

Some of the viruses may cause malignant neoplasms. These include Kaposi's sarcoma (KS), associated with a fairly newly recognised herpesvirus termed human herpesvirus type 8 (HHV-8); lymphomas (mainly non-Hodgkin type) associated with Epstein-Barr virus (EBV);

Table 3 WHO Classification of Oral Lesions in HIV/AIDS

Group I **Lesions strongly associated with HIV infection**	Group II **Lesions less commonly associated with HIV infection**	Group III **Lesions possibly associated with HIV infection**
Candidosis	Atypical ulceration (oropharyngeal)	A miscellany of rare diseases
Erythematous	Idiopathic thrombocytopenic purpura	
Thrush (pseudomembranous)	Salivary gland diseases	
Hairy leukoplakia (EBV)	Dry mouth	
HIV-gingivitis	Unilateral or bilateral swelling of major	
Necrotizing ulcerative gingivitis	salivary glands	
HIV-periodontitis.	Viral infections (other than EBV)	
Kaposi's sarcoma	Cytomegalovirus	
Non-Hodgkin's lymphoma	Herpes simplex virus	
	Human papillomavirus (HPV) (warty-like lesions): condyloma acuminatum, focal epithelial hyperplasia and verruca vulgaris.	
	Varicella-zoster virus: herpes zoster and varicella	

and cervical or anal carcinomas associated with human papillomaviruses (HPV).

Other important features of HIV/AIDS include anorexia, diarrhoea, wasting, dementia and other cerebral syndromes, and autoimmune phenomena such as blood platelet damage leading to thrombocytopenia and a bleeding tendency.

The prognosis of HIV/AIDS has been poor although antiretroviral therapy can result in significant control, and there are rare patients who show remarkable genetic resistance.

OROFACIAL FEATURES

The most common orofacial features of HIV/AIDS are cervical lymph node enlargement (Chapter 8) candidosis (candidiasis) and hairy leukoplakia (Figs. 2 and 3), but ulcers of various aetiologies (Chapter 2, Fig. 6), necrotising gingivitis, accelerated periodontitis, Kaposi's sarcoma, lymphomas and salivary gland disease are also seen (Table 3). The lesions are not absolutely specific for HIV infection and may occur in other immunocompromised groups. Most oral lesions occur in HIV-infected patients when the CD4 cell count is low and thus reflect the immunocompromised state of the patient.

The prevalence of most of these lesions has been decreasing following the advent of therapy with protease inhibitors, but HPV-related lesions and salivary gland complications appear to have increased, and lipodystrophy has appeared as a new adverse effect from protease inhibitors, along with various other orofacial sequelae (see below and Table 4).

DIAGNOSIS OF HIV INFECTION

Considerable compassion is called for in the management of HIV-infected persons. HIV infection is a catastrophic diagnosis since it impacts on virtually all aspects of the person's life as well as eventually possibly resulting in unpleasant, painful and incapacitating illnesses and their treatment. Confidentiality must be maintained at all times and the patient's consent and views always sought, including when considering informing other health care workers of any details about the person involved.

At the early stage there may be no detectable antibody production and thus testing the serum for HIV antibodies (serotesting) can lead to a false negative result. Only sophisticated and uncommonly used tests for HIV nucleic acid will detect the virus at this stage. Eventually, usually before six weeks, the serum antibodies to HIV become detectable.

The Enzyme-Linked ImmunoSorbent Assay (ELISA) for HIV p24 antibodies is the main serological test used but must be repeated and may need to be confirmed by a western blot test. False positive test reactions are known but rare.

MANAGEMENT

Complications of HIV/AIDS need treatment; this is mainly the treatment of opportunistic infections. Suppression, but not abolition, of the underlying HIV infection has become available following the development of anti-retroviral drugs. The first anti-retroviral agents included the nucleoside inhibitors of the HIV reverse transcriptase enzyme, zidovudine (ZDI sometimes termed AZT), didanosine (dideoxyinosine, ddI), and dideoxycytidine (ddC zalcitabine). Newer drugs include lamivudine (3TC) and stavudine (d4T) and the non-nucleoside reverse transcriptase inhibitors (delaviradine and nevaripine) (Table 4). The introduction of protease inhibitors (PIs), such as saquinavir, indinavir, ritonavir and nelfinavir proved to be a major advance. However, antiretroviral resistance is increasing, and a wide range of interactions can arise between protease inhibitors and other drugs, principally as a result of their metabolism by the same hepatic cytochrome P450 isoforms (Table 5). Entry inhibitors are the latest advance.

Highly active antiretroviral therapies (HAART) — combination therapy of a protease inhibitor with a reverse transcriptase inhibitor — reduce the incidence of infections and extend life substantially. Unfortunately, these agents are expensive. Some may produce oral adverse effects. Erythema multiforme and toxic epidermal necrolysis are especially well recognized as reactions to sulfonamides and to antiretroviral agents. Oral lichenoid reactions have been described relating to zidovudine use. Didanosine has also produced erythema multiforme and not unusually induces xerostomia. One of the more noticeable orofacial features of protease inhibitor use is swelling in the parotid region attributed to parotid lipomatosis as part of drug-induced lipodystrophy in which there is also dyslipidaemia and facial lipoatrophy.

Taste abnormalities are common with the protease inhibitors and oral and perioral paraesthesia can be a disturbing adverse effect.

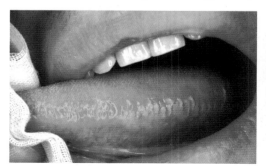

Figure 2. Candidosis in AIDS

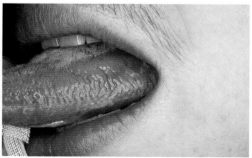

Figure 3. Hairy leukoplakia

Table 4 Antiretroviral drugs

Type	Generic name	Trade name	Possible orofacial adverse effects	Systemic main adverse effects
Nucleoside reverse transcriptase inhibitors (NRTIs)	Emtricitabine	Emtriva	Not recorded	Pruritus Nausea Diarrhoea Bone marrow suppression Lactic acidosis
	Zidovudine (azidothymidine) AZT ZDV	Retrovir	Erythema multiforme Hyperpigmentation	Nausea Diarrhoea Bone marrow suppression Lactic acidosis Myopathy
	Didanosine DDI	Videx	Erythema multiforme Xerostomia	Nausea Diarrhoea Lactic acidosis Pancreatitis Liver damage Peripheral neuropathy Retinal damage
	Zalcitabine DDC	Hivid	Erythema multiforme Ulcers	Lactic acidosis Pancreatitis Nausea Diarrhoea Liver damage
	Abacavir ABC	Ziagen	Erythema multiforme	Lactic acidosis Nausea Diarrhoea Life-threatening rash
	Lamivudine 3TC	Epivir	Xerostomia	Nausea Diarrhoea Pancreatitis Liver damage
	Stavudine D4T	Zerit	–	Neuro-psychiatric reactions Liver damage
Non-nucleoside reverse transcriptase inhibitors (NNRTIs)	Nevirapine	Viramune	Erythema multiforme Ulcers	Induces liver drug-metabolizing enzymes Liver damage
	Efavirenz	Sustiva	Erythema multiforme	Interferes with liver drug-metabolizing enzymes Neuro-psychiatric reactions
	Delavirdine	Rescriptor Not licensed in UK	Erythema multiforme	Inhibits liver drug-metabolizing enzymes
Protease inhibitors (PIs)	Indinavir IDV	Crixivan	Cheilitis Lipodystrophy Xerostomia Taste disturbance	Interferes with liver drug-metabolizing enzymes Nephrolithiasis Oesophagitis Haemolysis Dyslipidaemia
	Nelfinavir NFV	Viracept	Lipodystrophy Xerostomia	Nausea Diarrhoea Interferes with liver drug-metabolizing enzymes Dyslipidaemia
	Amprenavir APV (also available as pro-drug Fosamprenavir)	Agenerase	Paraesthesia Lipodystrophy	Interferes with liver drug-metabolizing enzymes Dyslipidaemia
	Ritonavir RTV (also available with lopinavir)	Norvir	Paraesthesia Lipodystrophy Xerostomia Taste disturbance Facial oedema	Nausea Diarrhoea Interferes with liver drug-metabolizing enzymes Flushing Dyslipidaemia
	Saquinavir SQV	Fortovase Invirase	Erythema multiforme Ulcers Lipodystrophy Xerostomia	Nausea Diarrhoea Interferes with liver drug-metabolizing enzymes Dyslipidaemia
Entry inhibitors	Enfuvirtide	Fuzeon	Sinusitis	Pancreatitis Neuropathy Hypersensitivity

Table 5 Potential interactions between HIV–protease inhibitors (PIs) and drugs used in the management of oral disease

Drugs used in oral health care	Examples	Comments on interactions with PIs	Probable clinical relevance
Antimycotics	Ketoconazole	Rise in levels of saquinavir and indinavir	Reduction in PI therapy may be required
	Fluconazole	Possible increase in levels of ritonavir or indinavir	Nil
	Itraconazole	Possible increase in levels of ritonavir or indinavir	Nil
Antibacterials	Sulfamethoxazole/ trimethoprim	Alteration in levels of sulfamethoxazole and/or trimethoprim	No change in drug therapies required
	Macrolides eg erythromycin and clindamycin	Possible interactions	Avoid or monitor for side-effects
	Metronidazole	Interaction with ritonavir	Disulfiram type reaction
Antihistamines	Astemizole or terfenadine	Cardiotoxic interactions	Avoid use of these antihistamines (possibly consider laratadine)
Immunosuppressives	Corticosteroids	Potential interaction(s)	Only use when clinically justified, monitor for drug side-effects
Benzodiazepines	Diazepam, midazolam, triazolam	Potential increased levels	Consider temazepam or lorazepam; monitor for adverse-effects and clinical efficacy
Anticonvulsants	Carbamazepine or phenytoin	Potential increased levels	Monitor for adverse-effects
Antidepressants	Tricyclic antidepressants or selective serotonin re-uptake inhibitors	Potential increased levels	Monitor for adverse-effects
Analgesics	Codeine, propoxyphene or piroxicam	Potential interference	Acetoaminophen and aspirin can be prescribed

MANAGEMENT OF OROFACIAL HEALTH

Oral hygiene should be maintained at a high standard and specific therapies used as indicated with due consideration of efficacy, oral and other adverse effects, drug interactions and cost.

Management of many of the lesions is facilitated if the carer has medical knowledge and always there must be collaboration with the physicians responsible for managing the patients.

Early treatment of oral candidosis is warranted not only because of the discomfort that may be caused by the lesions but also because the foci may act as reservoirs of organisms for local spread of disease particularly to the oesophagus. Antifungal prophylaxis should also be considered.

Treatment of oral hairy leukoplakia is not usually required but the condition often resolves with aciclovir or other agents active against EBV, or with anti-retroviral agents.

Oral KS lesions are often managed with topical tretinoin gel, intralesional vinblastine, or systemic chemotherapy (daunorubicin, oloxorubicin, paclitaxel or interferon) if there are extraoral lesions in addition.

Chemotherapy is required for treatment of lymphomas.

Granulocyte colony stimulating factor or thalidomide may be helpful in aphthous-like non-specific ulceration.

Akintoye SO, Greenberg MS. Recurrent aphthous stomatitis. Dent Clin North Am. 2005;49:31-47

Bsoul SA, Huber MA, Terezhalmy GT. Squamous cell carcinoma of the oral tissues: a comprehensive review for oral healthcare providers. J Contemp Dent Pract. 2005 15;6:1-16.

Clark GT, Minakuchi H, Lotaif AC. Orofacial pain and sensory disorders in the elderly. Dent Clin North Am. 2005;49:343-62.

Hentschel K, Capobianco DJ, Dodick DW. Facial pain. Neurologist. 2005;11:244-9.

Lodi G, Scully C, Carrozzo M, Griffiths M, Sugerman PB, Thongprasom K. Current controversies in oral lichen planus: report of an international consensus meeting. Part 2. Clinical management and malignant transformation. Oral Surg Oral Med Oral Pathol Oral Radiol Endod. 2005;100:164-78.

Noonan VL, Kabani S. Diagnosis and management of suspicious lesions of the oral cavity. Otolaryngol Clin North Am. 2005;38:21-35,

Okeson JP (Ed). Orofacial Pain: Guidelines for Assessment, Diagnosis, and Management 2005. Quintessence.

Porter SR, Scully C, Hegarty A. An update of the etiology and management of xerostomia.Oral Surg Oral Med Oral Pathol Oral Radiol Endod.; 2004; 97: 28-46.

Reichart PA, Philipsen HP. Oral erythroplakia--a review. Oral Oncol. 2005;41:551-61.

Reznik DA. Oral manifestations of HIV disease.Top HIV Med. 2005;13:143-8.

Sardella A, Lodi G, Demarosi F, Bez C, Cassano S, Carrassi A. Burning mouth syndrome: a retrospective study investigating spontaneous remission and response to treatments. Oral Dis. 2006;12:152-5.

Sciubba JJ, Goldenberg D. Oral complications of radiotherapy. Lancet Oncol. 2006;7:175-83.

Scully C, Epstein J, Sonis, S. Oral mucositis; A challenging complication of radiotherapy, chemotherapy, and radiochemotherapy: Part 2, diagnosis and management of mucositis. Head and Neck. 2004; 26: 77-84.

Scully C, Flint S, Porter SR, Moos K. *"Atlas of Oral and Maxillofacial Diseases"*. (2004) Taylor and Francis, London.

Scully C, Gorsky M, Lozada-Nur F. The diagnosis and management of recurrent aphthous stomatitis- a consensus approach. Journal of American Dental Association. 2003;134; 200-207.

Scully C, Rosenberg M. Halitosis. Dental Update 2003; 30; 205-210.

Scully C. *Oral and Maxillofacial Medicine.*(2004). Wright, Edinburgh

Scully, C, Boyle P. The role of the dental team in preventing and diagnosing cancer; Dental Update 2005; 32: 204-212.

Scully, C. Aphthous ulceration. New England Journal of Medicine. 2006; 355: 41-48.

Siccoli MM, Bassetti CL, Sandor PS. Facial pain: clinical differential diagnosis. Lancet Neurol. 2006; 5:257-67.

WEBLINKS

Reliable sites that contain abundant information-

Mayo Clinic
http://www.mayoclinic.com/health/dental/DE99999

National Institute of Dental and Craniofacial Research
http://www.nidcr.nih.gov/

emedicine
http://www.emedicine.com/